AF491158

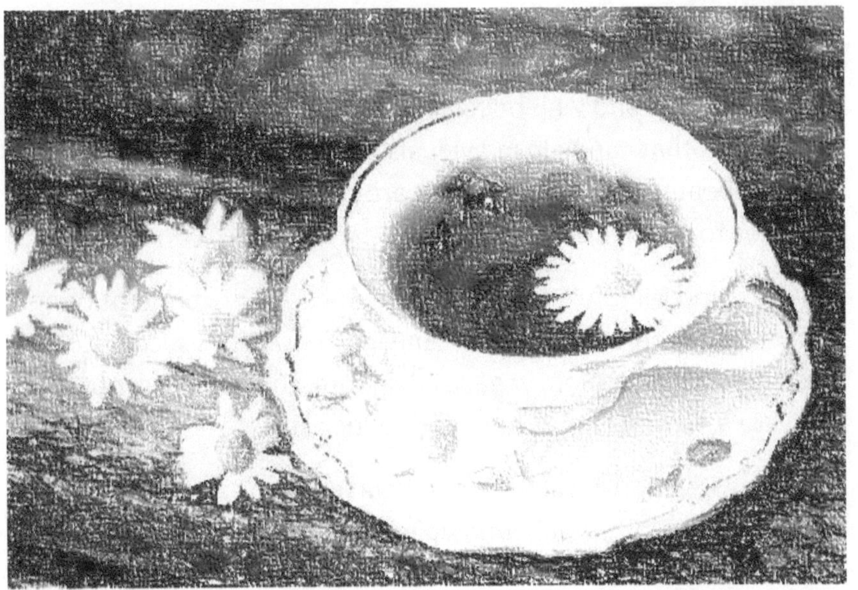

A Beautiful Life

Living a beautiful life with Irritable Bowel Syndrome (IBS) is possible, despite the challenges it may present. While IBS can impact daily life and well-being, there are strategies and approaches that can help individuals find joy, fulfillment, and a sense of beauty in their lives. Here are some perspectives and practices to consider:

Self-Care and Mindfulness: Prioritize self-care activities that bring you joy and promote relaxation. Engage in practices such as mindfulness meditation, yoga, or deep breathing exercises to cultivate a sense of inner calm and reduce stress.

Nurturing Relationships: Surround yourself with supportive and understanding individuals who uplift and inspire you. Build a network of friends, family, or support groups who can offer encouragement, empathy, and a listening ear.

Gratitude and Positive Mindset: Cultivate a gratitude practice by focusing on the positive aspects of your life. Recognize and appreciate the small moments of joy, achievements, and blessings that come your way. Adopting a positive mindset can help shift your perspective and enhance your overall well-being.

Pursue Passion and Hobbies: Explore activities or hobbies that bring you fulfillment and happiness. Engage in creative outlets, sports, arts, or any activity that allows you to express yourself and find a sense of purpose and enjoyment.

Balanced Lifestyle: Strive for balance in all areas of your life. Prioritize healthy eating habits, regular exercise, sufficient sleep, and stress management techniques. Creating a well-rounded lifestyle can support your overall health and help manage IBS symptoms.

Seek Support and Education: Stay informed about the latest research and information on IBS. Connect with reputable resources, such as healthcare professionals, reputable websites, or IBS organizations, to expand your knowledge and understanding of the condition. Seeking support and education can empower you to make informed decisions and navigate the challenges of living with IBS.

Practice Flexibility and Adaptability: IBS symptoms can be unpredictable, and it's important to be flexible and adapt to the ebb and flow of your condition. Embrace a mindset of acceptance and be kind to yourself during flare-ups or challenging times. Seek alternative solutions or adjustments to daily routines when needed.

Remember, living a beautiful life with IBS is about finding joy, embracing self-care, nurturing relationships, and cultivating a positive mindset. While IBS may present challenges, it doesn't define your entire life. By adopting a holistic approach, prioritizing self-care, and seeking support, you can create a fulfilling and beautiful life, even with IBS.

About the Author

Dr. Emily Anderson is a distinguished expert in the field of gastroenterology, specializing in the management and treatment of Irritable Bowel Syndrome (IBS). With a career spanning several decades, Dr. Anderson has dedicated her life to unraveling the complexities of IBS and helping individuals overcome the challenges associated with this chronic condition.

Drawing upon her extensive experience and expertise, Dr. Anderson has conducted numerous tests, therapy sessions, and cutting-edge research studies aimed at advancing the understanding and treatment of IBS. Her commitment to staying at the forefront of medical knowledge has allowed her to provide the most up-to-date and evidence-based solutions to her patients.

As a highly respected professor, Dr. Anderson has served as a mentor and educator to aspiring gastroenterologists, sharing her wealth of knowledge and fostering the next generation of experts in the field. She has contributed to various medical journals, authored several research papers, and presented at numerous national and international conferences, earning her recognition as a leading authority on IBS.

Dr. Anderson's genuine compassion and dedication to patient care have been instrumental in transforming the lives of countless individuals suffering from IBS. Through her private practice, she has helped patients regain control over their symptoms and improve their overall quality of life. Her patient-centric approach, coupled with her ability to effectively communicate complex medical information, has made her a trusted source of guidance and support.

"The IBS Solution: Empowering Yourself to Overcome Irritable Bowel Syndrome" is Dr. Anderson's groundbreaking book, offering a comprehensive and empowering guide for individuals seeking to overcome the challenges of IBS. In this book, she combines her clinical expertise, latest research insights, and practical strategies to provide readers with a roadmap to understanding their condition, managing symptoms, and reclaiming their lives. Dr. Anderson's compassionate approach, combined with her expertise, offers readers the tools and knowledge needed to take control of their health and find relief from the burdens of IBS.

Dr. Emily Anderson's contributions to the field of gastroenterology and her unwavering commitment to improving the lives of individuals with IBS have solidified her reputation as a respected authority. Her work continues to inspire hope and empower patients to overcome the challenges of IBS, offering a path toward a brighter and healthier future.

IBS

Book Summary: "The IBS Solution: Empowering Yourself to Overcome Irritable Bowel Syndrome" by Dr. Emily Anderson

"The IBS Solution: Empowering Yourself to Overcome Irritable Bowel Syndrome" written by Dr. Emily Anderson is a comprehensive guidebook that offers practical strategies, evidence-based insights, and empowering advice for individuals seeking to manage and overcome Irritable Bowel Syndrome (IBS).

In this book, Dr. Emily Anderson, a renowned expert in gastroenterology, provides a clear and compassionate understanding of IBS, its symptoms, and its impact on daily life. Drawing from her years of experience in treating patients with IBS, she demystifies the condition and offers hope to those seeking relief.

"The IBS Solution" takes a holistic approach to managing IBS, recognizing that every individual's experience with the condition is unique. Dr. Anderson explores the potential causes and triggers of IBS, including the role of gut health, diet, and stress. She emphasizes the importance of accurate diagnosis and encourages readers to work closely with healthcare professionals to develop a personalized treatment plan.

Throughout the book, Dr. Anderson addresses the various aspects of managing IBS, including dietary modifications, stress reduction techniques, and lifestyle adjustments. She explains the science behind different treatment approaches and offers practical tips for implementing them effectively.

One of the key strengths of "The IBS Solution" is Dr. Anderson's focus on empowering readers to take an active role in their own healing journey. She provides tools and strategies to help readers advocate for themselves, communicate effectively with healthcare providers, and track their symptoms to identify patterns and triggers.

The book also covers the emotional aspects of living with IBS. Dr. Anderson discusses the impact of stress, anxiety, and depression on IBS symptoms and provides practical guidance on managing emotions and improving overall well-being.

"The IBS Solution" goes beyond the traditional medical approaches and explores complementary therapies and alternative treatments that may be beneficial for some individuals. Dr. Anderson discusses the potential benefits of probiotics, herbal supplements, and mind-body practices, providing a well-rounded perspective on treatment options.

Written in a conversational and empathetic tone, "The IBS Solution" aims to empower readers with knowledge, support, and practical tools to overcome the challenges posed by IBS. It serves as a valuable resource for individuals with IBS, their loved ones, and healthcare professionals seeking a comprehensive understanding of the condition.

By combining scientific insights with real-life experiences and patient stories, Dr. Emily Anderson offers a roadmap for those seeking to take control of their IBS and lead a fulfilling life. "The IBS Solution" is an invaluable companion for anyone navigating the complexities of living with IBS and striving for long-term symptom relief and improved quality of life.

THE IBS SOLUTION: EMPOWERING YOURSELF TO OVERCOME IRRITABLE BOWEL SYNDROME

Dr. Emily Anderson

CONTENTS

INTRODUCTION

Irritable Bowel Syndrome (IBS) is a chronic condition that affects millions of people worldwide. Characterized by a range of uncomfortable gastrointestinal symptoms such as abdominal pain, bloating, diarrhea, and constipation, IBS can significantly impact an individual's quality of life, leading to physical discomfort, emotional distress, and limitations in daily activities. For those living with IBS, the journey to finding relief and effectively managing symptoms can be both frustrating and overwhelming.

In the face of such challenges, a wealth of information, resources, and strategies have emerged to empower individuals with IBS to take control of their condition, make informed decisions, and ultimately improve their well-being. This book serves as a comprehensive guide, providing a wealth of knowledge, practical tools, and empathetic support to help individuals navigate the complexities of IBS and empower themselves to overcome its impact.

Within the pages of this book, you will find insights from renowned experts, real-life stories from individuals who have successfully managed their IBS, and evidence-based strategies that have proven effective in the field. We will explore the diverse aspects of living with IBS, including its various subtypes, the underlying causes and contributing factors, and the potential triggers that can exacerbate symptoms. Through a holistic lens, we will delve into the role of diet and nutrition, exercise and physical activity, stress management techniques, and the importance of sleep in managing IBS.

Understanding that each person's experience with IBS is unique, we will address the importance of self-advocacy, open communication with healthcare professionals, and the importance of building a support network to navigate the challenges and uncertainties that often accompany this condition. We will delve into the emotional impact of IBS, exploring the interconnectedness between stress, anxiety, and symptoms, and offering practical approaches to managing emotional well-being.

Recognizing that there is no one-size-fits-all solution, we will explore a range of medical treatments, medications, and complementary therapies that have shown promise in alleviating IBS symptoms. Whether it's exploring the potential benefits of probiotics, herbal supplements, or mind-body practices, this book aims to provide a comprehensive understanding of the available options and empower individuals to make informed choices that align with their unique needs and preferences.

Throughout these pages, we hope to instill a sense of hope, encouragement, and empowerment. We want to remind you that while living with IBS can be challenging, it does not define who you are or your ability to lead a fulfilling life. By equipping you with knowledge, practical strategies, and a supportive community, we aim to empower you to take control of your IBS, manage symptoms effectively, and live a life that is not defined by your condition.

We invite you to embark on this journey of self-discovery and empowerment, as we navigate the complexities of Irritable Bowel Syndrome together. Let this book be your guide, your companion, and your source of inspiration as you embark on the path toward improved well-being and a balanced life, free from the constraints of IBS.

When living with Irritable Bowel Syndrome (IBS), individuals may encounter several significant challenges that can impact their daily lives. Here are some of the most common problems faced by people with IBS:

1. Physical Symptoms: The physical symptoms associated with IBS, such as abdominal pain, bloating, diarrhea, and constipation, can be uncomfortable and disruptive. These symptoms can vary in severity and frequency, making it difficult for individuals to engage in daily activities, work, or socialize without concern for potential flare-ups or discomfort.
2. Emotional Impact: IBS can have a profound emotional impact on individuals. Dealing with chronic pain and unpredictable symptoms can lead to feelings of frustration, anxiety, and depression. The uncertainty of when symptoms may arise and the impact they may have on daily life can significantly affect a person's mental well-being and overall quality of life.
3. Impact on Social Life: IBS can pose challenges in social situations. Individuals may feel anxious about attending events, going out to eat, or traveling, fearing that their symptoms may worsen or become embarrassing. This can lead to social isolation, as individuals may withdraw from social activities to avoid potential discomfort or embarrassment.
4. Impact on Work and Productivity: The symptoms of IBS can interfere with work and productivity. Frequent bathroom breaks, abdominal pain, and difficulty concentrating can make it challenging to perform optimally in the workplace. Some individuals may face limitations or difficulties in their careers due to their condition, which can cause frustration and impact their professional growth.
5. Dietary Restrictions and Challenges: Many individuals with IBS find that certain foods trigger or worsen their symptoms. This can lead to the need for dietary

modifications, such as following a low FODMAP diet or avoiding specific food groups. Adhering to dietary restrictions can be challenging, both in terms of meal planning and navigating social situations that involve food.

6. Difficulty in Diagnosis and Treatment: Diagnosing IBS can be a complex process, as there is no specific test for the condition. Individuals may undergo numerous medical tests and consultations before receiving a diagnosis, which can be frustrating and time-consuming. Additionally, finding an effective treatment plan tailored to the individual's unique symptoms and triggers may require trial and error, leading to further frustration and uncertainty.

7. Lack of Understanding and Support: IBS is an invisible condition, meaning that individuals may not appear sick to others. This can lead to a lack of understanding and empathy from friends, family, and even healthcare professionals. Some individuals may struggle to explain their symptoms or feel invalidated, which can further impact their emotional well-being and sense of support.

Despite these challenges, it's important to remember that there are strategies, treatments, and support systems available to help individuals with IBS manage their condition and improve their quality of life. By seeking guidance from healthcare professionals, finding support from understanding individuals or support groups, and implementing self-care practices, individuals with IBS can navigate these challenges and find ways to live fulfilling lives while managing their symptoms.

People suffering from Irritable Bowel Syndrome (IBS) can experience a range of physical and emotional challenges that significantly impact their daily lives. Here are some ways in which individuals with IBS may suffer:

1. Physical Discomfort: Individuals with IBS often experience physical symptoms that can be uncomfortable and painful. These may include abdominal pain, cramping, bloating, gas, diarrhea, constipation, or a combination of these symptoms. The severity and frequency of symptoms can vary, but they can significantly interfere with daily activities and overall well-being.
2. Limitations in Activities: The unpredictable nature of IBS symptoms can lead to limitations in activities. Individuals may feel hesitant to engage in social events, travel, or participate in certain physical activities due to concerns about symptom flare-ups. This can lead to a decreased quality of life and feelings of isolation or missing out on experiences.
3. Emotional Distress: IBS can cause emotional distress, including increased stress, anxiety, and depression. The constant uncertainty of when symptoms may occur and the impact they may have on daily life can take a toll on mental well-being. The emotional burden of dealing with a chronic condition can lead to frustration, irritability, and a decreased sense of overall happiness.
4. Disruption of Daily Routine: The presence of IBS symptoms can disrupt daily routines and activities. Frequent visits to the bathroom, sudden urgency, or prolonged periods of discomfort can interfere with work, school, and personal commitments. This disruption can lead to feelings of frustration, a sense of loss of control, and difficulties in planning and maintaining a consistent routine.
5. Dietary Challenges: Many individuals with IBS experience food sensitivities or triggers that can exacerbate symptoms. This often necessitates dietary modifications, such as avoiding certain foods or following specialized diets like the low FODMAP diet. Adhering to dietary restrictions can be challenging and may require careful meal planning, label

reading, and navigating social situations that revolve around food.
6. Impact on Relationships: IBS can strain relationships with friends, family, and romantic partners. The need to accommodate IBS symptoms and the limitations it may impose on social activities can create tension or misunderstandings. The emotional and physical toll of the condition may also lead to decreased intimacy or strained connections within relationships.
7. Lack of Understanding and Support: Due to the invisible nature of IBS, individuals may face a lack of understanding and empathy from others. The unpredictable and fluctuating nature of symptoms can make it difficult for others to comprehend the impact on daily life. This lack of understanding and support can exacerbate feelings of isolation and contribute to the emotional burden of the condition.

It is important for individuals with IBS to seek appropriate medical care, establish a strong support system, and explore coping strategies to help manage symptoms and address the emotional impact of the condition. By finding effective treatment strategies, building understanding relationships, and prioritizing self-care, individuals with IBS can work towards improving their overall well-being and finding ways to cope with the challenges they face.

While there is no one-size-fits-all solution for managing Irritable Bowel Syndrome (IBS), there are various strategies and approaches that can help individuals find relief and improve their quality of life. Here are some ways people can address and manage their IBS:

1. Seek Professional Guidance: Consult with a healthcare professional, such as a gastroenterologist or primary care physician, who specializes in digestive disorders. They can

help diagnose your condition, rule out other potential causes, and develop a personalized treatment plan tailored to your specific symptoms and needs.

2. Educate Yourself: Learn about IBS to better understand your condition and potential triggers. Knowledge empowers you to make informed decisions about your lifestyle, diet, and treatment options. Reliable sources such as reputable medical websites, books, and support groups can provide valuable information.

3. Dietary Modifications: Work with a registered dietitian who specializes in digestive disorders to identify trigger foods and develop a suitable eating plan. Consider exploring diets like the low FODMAP diet, which focuses on reducing specific carbohydrates that can worsen IBS symptoms. Keep a food diary to track your symptoms in relation to your diet.

4. Stress Reduction: Practice stress management techniques such as mindfulness meditation, deep breathing exercises, yoga, or engaging in activities that promote relaxation. Reducing stress levels can help minimize the impact of stress on IBS symptoms.

5. Regular Exercise: Engage in regular physical activity, such as walking, swimming, or yoga, as it can help alleviate symptoms and improve overall well-being. Aim for at least 30 minutes of moderate exercise most days of the week, but listen to your body and adjust intensity as needed.

6. Medications and Supplements: Discuss medication options with your healthcare provider. They may recommend over-the-counter medications for symptom relief or prescribe specific medications targeted at IBS symptoms, such as antispasmodics or medications that regulate bowel movements. Some individuals may find relief from certain supplements, such as peppermint oil or probiotics, but it's

important to consult with your healthcare provider before starting any supplements.

7. Support Network: Connect with others who have IBS through support groups, online forums, or local community groups. Sharing experiences, tips, and emotional support can be valuable in navigating the challenges of IBS. Consider seeking therapy or counseling to address the emotional impact of living with a chronic condition.
8. Lifestyle Adjustments: Identify and modify lifestyle factors that may exacerbate your symptoms. This may include improving sleep habits, implementing relaxation techniques, and maintaining a consistent daily routine.
9. Experiment and Track: Keep a symptom diary to identify patterns and triggers for your symptoms. Experiment with different strategies, such as stress reduction techniques, dietary changes, and medications, to see what works best for you. It may take time to find the right combination of approaches.
10. Be Patient and Kind to Yourself: Managing IBS can be a journey of trial and error. Be patient with yourself and practice self-compassion. It may take time to find the right strategies and treatments that work for you. Remember that everyone's experience with IBS is unique, and finding a personalized approach is key.

By taking a proactive approach, seeking professional guidance, and implementing lifestyle modifications, individuals can effectively manage their IBS symptoms and improve their overall well-being. Remember to consult with healthcare professionals to develop a tailored plan that meets your specific needs and goals.

While it's important to acknowledge the potential impact of stress and the mind-body connection on Irritable Bowel Syndrome (IBS), it is essential to approach this topic with caution and critical thinking. While there is evidence to suggest that stress and psychological factors can influence IBS symptoms, it is crucial to recognize that IBS is a complex medical condition with various contributing factors, including physiological, genetic, and environmental factors.

The concept of the law of attraction, which suggests that positive thinking and visualization can influence one's health outcomes, is not based on scientific evidence and should be approached with skepticism. It is important to prioritize evidence-based approaches to managing IBS symptoms and consult with healthcare professionals who specialize in digestive disorders.

However, it is worth noting that psychological interventions, such as cognitive-behavioral therapy (CBT), relaxation techniques, and mindfulness-based stress reduction, have shown promise in helping individuals with IBS manage their symptoms by addressing stress and improving coping strategies. These approaches focus on evidence-based psychological techniques rather than metaphysical concepts like the law of attraction.

If you are interested in exploring the mind-body connection in relation to IBS, it is recommended to consult with a healthcare professional or therapist who specializes in this area. They can provide guidance and support based on scientific evidence and help you develop strategies to manage stress, improve your overall well-being, and effectively cope with IBS symptoms.

THE BOOK'S PURPOSE

Welcome to "The IBS Solution: Empowering Yourself to Overcome Irritable Bowel Syndrome." In this book, Dr. Emily Anderson, a distinguished expert in the field of gastroenterology, shares her expertise, research, and experiences to provide you with a comprehensive guide to understanding and managing Irritable Bowel Syndrome (IBS).

The primary purpose of this book is to empower individuals who suffer from IBS by providing them with practical knowledge, effective strategies, and a sense of control over their condition. Dr. Anderson's goal is to help you navigate the challenges of IBS and develop a personalized approach to managing your symptoms, improving your overall well-being, and reclaiming your life.

Dr. Emily Anderson brings decades of experience and a wealth of knowledge to this book. As a leading authority on IBS, she has dedicated her career to unraveling the complexities of this condition and finding innovative solutions for her patients. Driven by her personal journey with IBS, she understands the physical and emotional impact it can have on individuals and the importance of effective management strategies.

Throughout her career, Dr. Anderson has conducted extensive research, collaborated with esteemed institutions, and actively participated in clinical trials and studies. Her commitment to staying at the forefront of medical knowledge ensures that the information provided in this book is based on the latest research findings and emerging theories.

Dr. Anderson's expertise extends beyond research and academia. She has successfully treated and helped numerous individuals overcome the challenges of IBS through her private practice. Her compassionate and patient-centered approach has earned her a reputation for providing comprehensive care and personalized treatment plans that address the unique needs of each individual.

By sharing her experiences, research, and insights, Dr. Anderson aims to empower you with the tools and knowledge needed to navigate your IBS journey effectively. Her expertise, combined with her genuine empathy, makes her a trusted source of guidance and support for those seeking relief from the burdens of IBS.

In the following chapters, Dr. Anderson will delve into various aspects of IBS, including its causes, symptoms, diagnosis, treatment options, lifestyle adjustments, coping strategies, and more. By the end of this book, you will have a comprehensive understanding of IBS and be equipped with practical tools to take charge of your health and well-being.

Remember, you are not alone in your journey. Dr. Anderson is here to provide you with the information, guidance, and support you need to overcome IBS and live a fulfilling life. Let's embark on this transformative journey together.

UNDERSTANDING IRRITABLE BOWEL SYNDROME

Irritable Bowel Syndrome (IBS) is a chronic gastrointestinal disorder that affects the large intestine (colon). It is characterized by a combination of various symptoms, including abdominal pain, bloating, gas, diarrhea, and constipation. Individuals with IBS often experience these symptoms in a recurrent and chronic manner, which can significantly impact their quality of life.

IBS is a common disorder, with a significant global prevalence. It affects people of all ages, although it tends to occur more frequently in young adults. It is estimated that up to 10-15% of the global population may be affected by IBS at some point in their lives. While IBS can affect both men and women, it tends to be more prevalent in women.

The exact cause of IBS is not fully understood, but it is believed to be a combination of various factors. Abnormal intestinal contractions and motility, which can lead to either diarrhea or constipation, play a role in IBS. Individuals with IBS may also have heightened sensitivity in their gut, leading to visceral hypersensitivity and amplified pain perception. Additionally, factors such as genetics, environmental triggers, and imbalances in the gut microbiota have been implicated in the development of IBS.

There are different subtypes of IBS based on predominant bowel habits. These include:

- IBS with constipation (IBS-C): Characterized by infrequent bowel movements and the presence of hard, lumpy stools.

- IBS with diarrhea (IBS-D): Characterized by frequent bowel movements, loose or watery stools, and a sense of urgency.
- Mixed IBS (IBS-M): Characterized by alternating episodes of constipation and diarrhea.

Each subtype presents with its own set of challenges and symptom patterns, requiring tailored approaches to management.

Various triggers and aggravating factors can worsen IBS symptoms. These include certain foods, such as those high in FODMAPs (fermentable carbohydrates), gluten, lactose, and spicy or fatty foods. Stress, anxiety, and emotional factors can also play a role in triggering or exacerbating symptoms. Other factors, such as hormonal changes, medications, and environmental triggers, may contribute to symptom flare-ups.

IBS can significantly impact an individual's quality of life. The symptoms of IBS can be disruptive, leading to physical discomfort, emotional distress, and limitations in daily activities. It can affect social interactions, work productivity, and overall well-being. Understanding the impact of IBS on quality of life is crucial in developing comprehensive management strategies.

By gaining a thorough understanding of what IBS is, its prevalence, causes, subtypes, triggers, and impact on quality of life, you will be better equipped to navigate the subsequent chapters, which will provide you with strategies for managing and overcoming the challenges posed by IBS.

Diagnosing IBS involves a comprehensive evaluation of symptoms, medical history, and physical examinations. There are specific criteria, known as the Rome criteria, that healthcare professionals use to diagnose IBS. Diagnostic tests, such as blood tests, stool tests, and imaging studies, may be performed to rule out other potential underlying causes of gastrointestinal symptoms. It is important to consult with a healthcare professional for an accurate diagnosis.

There are several misconceptions and myths surrounding IBS. It is often dismissed or misunderstood as a purely psychological condition or simply a result of stress. However, IBS is a real medical condition with physical manifestations. Dispelling these misconceptions is crucial for proper understanding and management of the condition.

IBS is considered a chronic condition, meaning it is ongoing and long-lasting. While there may be periods of symptom remission, it is important to recognize that IBS is a chronic disorder that requires ongoing management and lifestyle adjustments.

Living with IBS can be challenging, and seeking support is essential. Connecting with support groups, online communities, and seeking guidance from healthcare professionals who specialize in IBS can provide valuable resources, understanding, and tools for managing the condition effectively.

DEFINITION AND EXPLANATION OF IBS

IBS stands for Irritable Bowel Syndrome. It is a common disorder that affects the large intestine (colon) and causes a variety of digestive symptoms. IBS is considered a functional gastrointestinal disorder, meaning that it affects the normal functioning of the digestive system without any visible signs of damage or disease.

The exact cause of IBS is not well understood, but it is believed to involve a combination of factors, including abnormalities in the gut-brain axis, changes in gut motility (the movement of the digestive tract), visceral hypersensitivity (increased sensitivity to pain in the intestines), and an imbalance of gut bacteria. Psychological factors such as stress, anxiety, and depression can also play a role in triggering or exacerbating symptoms.

The primary symptoms of IBS include abdominal pain or discomfort, bloating, gas, and changes in bowel habits, such as diarrhea, constipation, or a combination of both. These symptoms may vary in severity and can occur in episodes or flare-ups. Some individuals with IBS may also experience other non-digestive symptoms like fatigue, sleep disturbances, and mood disorders.

Diagnosing IBS involves ruling out other medical conditions that may cause similar symptoms. There are no specific tests to definitively diagnose IBS, but doctors may perform a physical examination, review the patient's medical history, and order certain tests to exclude other possible causes.

Treatment for IBS aims to manage and alleviate symptoms rather than cure the condition. It typically involves a combination of lifestyle modifications, dietary changes, stress management techniques, and, in some cases, medications to relieve specific symptoms like pain, diarrhea, or constipation. Dietary adjustments may include avoiding certain trigger foods, increasing fiber intake, and adopting a low-FODMAP diet, which limits the consumption of fermentable carbohydrates that can worsen symptoms in some people.

While IBS can be a chronic condition, its impact on daily life can be minimized through symptom management strategies and by working closely with healthcare professionals to develop an individualized treatment plan. It's important for individuals with IBS to understand their triggers and adopt a proactive approach to managing their symptoms.

PREVALENCE AND DEMOGRAPHICS

IBS is a common gastrointestinal disorder that affects people of all ages, although it tends to be more prevalent in young adults. The exact prevalence of IBS varies depending on the population studied and the diagnostic criteria used. Estimates suggest that IBS affects around 10-15% of the global population.

In terms of demographics, IBS appears to be more common in women than in men. Women are estimated to be twice as likely as men to be diagnosed with IBS. The reason for this gender difference is not entirely clear and may be influenced by hormonal factors, differences in pain perception, and societal or cultural factors.

IBS can occur in people of all ethnic backgrounds, although some studies have suggested that certain populations may have a higher prevalence. For example, studies have reported a higher prevalence of IBS in Western countries compared to Eastern countries, but these differences may be influenced by variations in diagnostic criteria and reporting.

1. Age: While IBS can occur at any age, it often begins in late adolescence or early adulthood. However, it can also develop in children and older adults. It is less common for IBS symptoms to first appear after the age of 50.
2. Impact on Quality of Life: IBS can significantly affect a person's quality of life, leading to decreased productivity, impaired social functioning, and emotional distress. The impact of IBS can vary from person to person, with some experiencing mild symptoms that do not significantly disrupt daily life, while others may have more severe symptoms that significantly impact their overall well-being.

3. Comorbidities: Individuals with IBS may have a higher likelihood of having other medical conditions alongside their IBS symptoms. For example, there is an association between IBS and conditions such as fibromyalgia, chronic fatigue syndrome, temporomandibular joint disorder (TMJ), and certain mental health disorders like anxiety and depression. It is important for healthcare providers to consider these potential comorbidities when managing IBS.

4. Psychological Factors: Psychological factors, such as stress, anxiety, and depression, can influence the onset and severity of IBS symptoms. It is not uncommon for individuals with IBS to experience heightened stress or anxiety related to their symptoms, which can create a vicious cycle of exacerbating digestive symptoms.

5. Diagnostic Challenges: Diagnosing IBS can be challenging due to its subjective nature and the absence of specific diagnostic tests. The Rome criteria, a set of standardized symptom-based criteria, are commonly used to diagnose IBS. However, the criteria have evolved over time, and different versions exist, which can contribute to variations in prevalence rates across studies.

It's important to remember that the prevalence and demographics of IBS can vary in different regions and populations. Research in this area continues to evolve, aiming to improve our understanding of the condition and provide better support and management strategies for individuals with IBS.

It's worth noting that IBS is a condition that often goes underreported, and many individuals with symptoms do not seek medical attention or receive a formal diagnosis. This can make it challenging to determine the exact prevalence and demographics of IBS accurately.

Overall, IBS is a widespread disorder that affects individuals of different ages, genders, and ethnic backgrounds. It is essential to raise awareness about the condition and promote understanding and support for individuals living with IBS.

CAUSES AND CONTRIBUTING FACTORS

The exact causes of IBS are not fully understood, but it is believed to involve a combination of factors. Here are some potential causes and contributing factors that have been identified:

1. Gut-Brain Axis Dysfunction: The gut and brain communicate bidirectionally through the gut-brain axis. Disruptions in this communication may contribute to the development of IBS. Stress, emotions, and psychological factors can influence gut function and sensitivity, leading to IBS symptoms.
2. Abnormal Gut Motility: The muscles in the digestive tract contract in a coordinated manner to move food through the intestines. In people with IBS, these contractions may be irregular or spasmodic, leading to changes in bowel habits. Some individuals may experience diarrhea-predominant IBS (IBS-D) with rapid movement of stool, while others may have constipation-predominant IBS (IBS-C) with slower transit.
3. Visceral Hypersensitivity: People with IBS often have heightened sensitivity or enhanced perception of pain and discomfort in the intestines. This means that normal intestinal sensations, such as gas or stool movement, can be perceived as painful or uncomfortable in individuals with IBS.
4. Intestinal Inflammation: Low-grade inflammation in the intestines has been observed in some individuals with IBS, particularly in those with post-infectious IBS (IBS-PI). Infections of the gastrointestinal tract, such as bacterial or viral gastroenteritis, can trigger IBS symptoms in susceptible individuals.

5. Altered Gut Microbiota: The gut is home to trillions of bacteria, collectively known as the gut microbiota. Imbalances in the composition of gut bacteria, termed dysbiosis, have been associated with IBS. It is thought that alterations in the gut microbiota may contribute to inflammation, increased gut permeability, and abnormal gut function seen in IBS.
6. Food Intolerances and Sensitivities: Certain types of food may trigger or worsen symptoms in individuals with IBS. Common culprits include fermentable carbohydrates known as FODMAPs (fermentable oligosaccharides, disaccharides, monosaccharides, and polyols). These substances can cause gas, bloating, and changes in bowel movements in susceptible individuals.
7. Genetic and Environmental Factors: There may be a genetic predisposition to developing IBS, as it tends to run in families. Environmental factors, such as early life stress, traumatic events, and childhood abuse, have been associated with an increased risk of developing IBS.

It's important to note that these factors are not mutually exclusive, and different individuals may have different combinations of contributing factors. Additionally, triggers for IBS symptoms can vary from person to person, and what worsens symptoms for one individual may not affect another.

Understanding the causes and contributing factors of IBS is crucial for developing effective treatment strategies and personalized approaches to managing the condition. However, more research is needed to fully elucidate the complex mechanisms underlying IBS.

RECOGNIZING IBS SYMPTOMS

Recognizing the symptoms of IBS is important for early detection and proper management of the condition. Here are the common symptoms associated with Irritable Bowel Syndrome (IBS):

1. Abdominal Pain or Discomfort: Recurring abdominal pain or discomfort is a hallmark symptom of IBS. The pain is typically located in the lower abdomen and may vary in intensity. It is often described as crampy or colicky in nature.
2. Changes in Bowel Habits: IBS can cause changes in bowel movements, leading to different patterns. These patterns may include:
    o Diarrhea-Predominant IBS (IBS-D): Frequent loose or watery stools occur, often accompanied by an urgent need to have a bowel movement.
    o Constipation-Predominant IBS (IBS-C): Bowel movements become infrequent, and stools may be hard, lumpy, or difficult to pass.
    o Mixed IBS (IBS-M): Alternating episodes of diarrhea and constipation are experienced.
    o Unsubtyped IBS (IBS-U): Symptoms do not clearly fit into any specific category.
3. Bloating and Excessive Gas: Many individuals with IBS experience bloating, which is a sensation of fullness or swelling in the abdomen. It may be accompanied by increased flatulence (passing gas).
4. Changes in Stool Appearance: Stool consistency and appearance can vary in IBS. Some individuals may notice mucus in their stool or have a feeling of incomplete evacuation after a bowel movement.

5. Abdominal Discomfort Relieved by Defecation: In IBS, the discomfort or pain in the abdomen often improves or resolves after a bowel movement.
6. Other Symptoms: Some people with IBS may experience additional symptoms, such as fatigue, sleep disturbances, urgency to urinate, a sense of incomplete bladder emptying, and non-specific backache.

It's important to note that the severity and frequency of these symptoms can vary among individuals with IBS. Symptoms may also fluctuate over time, with periods of remission and flare-ups.

If you suspect you may have IBS or are experiencing persistent gastrointestinal symptoms, it is recommended to consult a healthcare professional for an accurate diagnosis. They will consider your medical history, perform a physical examination, and may order tests to rule out other possible causes of your symptoms.

COMMON SYMPTOMS EXPERIENCED BY IBS SUFFERERS

Common symptoms experienced by individuals with Irritable Bowel Syndrome (IBS) include:

1. Abdominal Pain or Discomfort: Recurring abdominal pain or discomfort is a primary symptom of IBS. The pain is typically characterized as cramping, colicky, or aching. It is often relieved or partially relieved after a bowel movement.
2. Altered Bowel Habits: IBS can cause changes in bowel movements, leading to different patterns:
    - Diarrhea: Some individuals experience frequent loose or watery stools. They may have an urgent need to have a bowel movement and may need to rush to the bathroom.
    - Constipation: Others may have infrequent bowel movements, with stools that are hard, lumpy, or difficult to pass. They may feel like they haven't fully emptied their bowels.
    - Mixed Bowel Habits: Some individuals experience alternating episodes of diarrhea and constipation. These alternating patterns can occur over weeks or months.
3. Bloating and Excessive Gas: Many people with IBS experience bloating, which is a feeling of fullness, tightness, or swelling in the abdomen. It is often accompanied by increased gas production and flatulence.
4. Abdominal Distension: The abdomen may appear visibly swollen or distended due to increased gas accumulation or bloating.

5. Mucus in Stool: Some individuals with IBS may notice the presence of mucus in their stools. While mucus in the stool is not unique to IBS, it can be a common occurrence in individuals with this condition.
6. Urgency and Incomplete Evacuation: Some people with IBS may experience a sense of urgency to have a bowel movement, with a feeling of needing to go immediately. Additionally, they may have a sensation of incomplete evacuation, feeling like there is more stool to pass even after having a bowel movement.
7. Fatigue and Sleep Disturbances: Chronic fatigue is common among individuals with IBS. Sleep disturbances, including insomnia or disrupted sleep patterns, can also be associated with IBS.
8. Anxiety and Depression: Psychological symptoms, such as anxiety and depression, are often observed in individuals with IBS. The relationship between IBS and these conditions is complex, with one potentially influencing the other.

It's important to note that not all individuals with IBS experience the same set of symptoms, and the severity and frequency of symptoms can vary. Additionally, some individuals may experience symptoms outside of the gastrointestinal tract, such as headaches, muscle pain, and urinary symptoms.

If you are experiencing persistent or bothersome gastrointestinal symptoms, it is advisable to consult with a healthcare professional for an accurate diagnosis and appropriate management strategies.

DIFFERENTIATING IBS FROM OTHER GASTROINTESTINAL DISORDERS

Differentiating Irritable Bowel Syndrome (IBS) from other gastrointestinal disorders can be challenging due to overlapping symptoms and the absence of specific diagnostic tests for IBS. However, healthcare professionals consider several factors to help distinguish IBS from other conditions. Here are some points to consider:

1. Diagnostic Criteria: IBS is typically diagnosed based on symptom-based criteria, such as the Rome criteria, which require the presence of specific symptoms for a specified duration. These criteria help differentiate IBS from other gastrointestinal disorders that may have distinct diagnostic criteria.
2. Absence of Alarm Symptoms: Alarm symptoms refer to warning signs that may indicate a more serious underlying condition. These symptoms include unexplained weight loss, rectal bleeding, anemia, fever, and a family history of gastrointestinal diseases like inflammatory bowel disease or colon cancer. The presence of alarm symptoms is an indication for further investigation to rule out other conditions.
3. Age of Onset: IBS can develop at any age, but it is more commonly diagnosed in young adults. On the other hand, certain gastrointestinal disorders, such as inflammatory bowel disease (Crohn's disease or ulcerative colitis), are more prevalent in younger individuals, while conditions like colon cancer are more common in older individuals. The age of onset can provide some clues for differentiation.
4. Inflammatory Markers: Inflammatory bowel diseases, such as Crohn's disease and ulcerative colitis, are characterized

by chronic inflammation of the digestive tract. Specific tests, such as blood tests for inflammatory markers (C-reactive protein, erythrocyte sedimentation rate) and stool tests for fecal calprotectin, can help identify inflammation and distinguish IBS from these inflammatory conditions.

5. Structural Abnormalities: Structural abnormalities in the digestive tract, such as strictures, tumors, or anatomical malformations, can cause symptoms similar to IBS. Imaging tests like colonoscopy, flexible sigmoidoscopy, or abdominal ultrasound can help identify such abnormalities and differentiate them from IBS.

6. Food Allergies/Intolerances: Some food allergies or intolerances, such as celiac disease (gluten intolerance) or lactose intolerance, can cause gastrointestinal symptoms similar to those of IBS. Specific diagnostic tests, such as blood tests for celiac disease antibodies or lactose intolerance breath tests, can help identify these conditions.

It is important to note that these points are general guidelines, and the diagnosis of IBS should be made by a qualified healthcare professional based on a comprehensive evaluation of the individual's symptoms, medical history, physical examination, and appropriate diagnostic tests.

If you are experiencing persistent gastrointestinal symptoms or are concerned about your health, it is recommended to consult a healthcare professional for an accurate diagnosis and appropriate management.

GETTING DIAGNOSED

Getting diagnosed with Irritable Bowel Syndrome (IBS) typically involves several steps. Here is a general outline of the diagnostic process:

1. Medical History: Your healthcare provider will start by taking a detailed medical history, including a discussion of your symptoms, their duration and frequency, and any factors that may worsen or alleviate them. They may also ask about your family history of gastrointestinal disorders.
2. Physical Examination: A physical examination will be conducted to assess your overall health and to check for any signs of other medical conditions that could be causing your symptoms.
3. Symptom Evaluation: Your healthcare provider will evaluate your symptoms based on the diagnostic criteria for IBS. The Rome criteria, which are commonly used, require the presence of specific symptoms for a defined duration. These criteria help establish if your symptoms are consistent with IBS.
4. Diagnostic Tests: While there is no specific test to definitively diagnose IBS, your healthcare provider may order certain tests to rule out other possible causes of your symptoms. These tests may include:
   - Blood Tests: Blood tests can help evaluate for certain conditions that may mimic IBS symptoms, such as celiac disease, thyroid disorders, or inflammatory markers.
   - Stool Tests: Stool tests can check for signs of infection, parasites, or other abnormalities that may be causing your symptoms.

- o Imaging Tests: In some cases, your healthcare provider may order imaging tests, such as colonoscopy, flexible sigmoidoscopy, or abdominal ultrasound, to evaluate the structure and condition of your digestive tract and rule out any structural abnormalities.
5. Elimination Diets: In certain situations, your healthcare provider may recommend an elimination diet to identify potential food triggers that worsen your symptoms. This may involve removing specific food groups, such as gluten or lactose, for a period of time and then gradually reintroducing them to assess their impact on your symptoms.

It's important to note that the diagnostic process may vary depending on your specific situation and the practices of your healthcare provider. It's crucial to communicate openly with your healthcare provider about your symptoms, concerns, and any questions you may have.

Remember, a proper diagnosis is important to ensure appropriate management and treatment of your symptoms. If you suspect you may have IBS or are experiencing persistent gastrointestinal symptoms, it is recommended to consult with a healthcare professional who can guide you through the diagnostic process and develop an individualized treatment plan.

THE DIAGNOSTIC PROCESS FOR IBS

The diagnostic process for Irritable Bowel Syndrome (IBS) typically involves a combination of medical history, symptom evaluation, and exclusion of other potential causes. Here is a general overview of the diagnostic process for IBS:

1. Medical History: Your healthcare provider will begin by taking a detailed medical history, which involves asking questions about your symptoms, their duration, and any factors that may worsen or alleviate them. They will also inquire about your medical history, family history of gastrointestinal disorders, and any relevant lifestyle or dietary factors.
2. Symptom Evaluation: Your healthcare provider will assess your symptoms based on established diagnostic criteria. The Rome criteria are commonly used, which require the presence of abdominal pain or discomfort for at least three days per month in the past three months, along with two or more of the following criteria: improvement with bowel movements, changes in stool frequency, or changes in stool consistency. Meeting these criteria helps support a diagnosis of IBS.
3. Exclusion of Other Conditions: To rule out other potential causes of your symptoms, your healthcare provider may order certain tests. These tests are primarily performed to exclude conditions that can mimic IBS symptoms, such as inflammatory bowel disease, celiac disease, thyroid disorders, or colon cancer. The specific tests ordered may vary depending on your symptoms, medical history, and individual factors.
    - Blood tests: Blood tests may be conducted to check for markers of inflammation, rule out celiac disease,

assess thyroid function, or evaluate for other potential underlying conditions.

- o Stool tests: Stool tests may be recommended to rule out infections, parasites, or signs of inflammation in the digestive tract.
- o Imaging tests: In some cases, imaging tests like colonoscopy, flexible sigmoidoscopy, or abdominal ultrasound may be performed to visualize the colon and rule out structural abnormalities or other gastrointestinal disorders.

4. Clinical Judgment: Your healthcare provider will use their clinical judgment to assess the overall pattern of your symptoms, evaluate the results of diagnostic tests, and make a diagnosis. They will consider the presence of typical IBS symptoms, the absence of alarm symptoms (such as rectal bleeding or unexplained weight loss), and the exclusion of other conditions.

It's important to note that there is no specific test that can definitively diagnose IBS. The diagnosis is primarily made based on the characteristic symptoms and the exclusion of other potential causes.

If you suspect you may have IBS or are experiencing persistent gastrointestinal symptoms, it is recommended to consult with a healthcare professional. They will guide you through the diagnostic process, evaluate your symptoms, and develop an appropriate management plan tailored to your specific needs.

MEDICAL TESTS AND EVALUATIONS

When evaluating a patient for Irritable Bowel Syndrome (IBS) or ruling out other potential causes of gastrointestinal symptoms, healthcare providers may recommend various medical tests and evaluations. While there is no specific test to definitively diagnose IBS, these tests help exclude other conditions and provide a comprehensive assessment. Here are some common tests and evaluations that may be performed:

1. Blood Tests: Blood tests can be used to assess various factors, including:
    - Complete blood count (CBC): Helps evaluate for anemia or signs of infection.
    - Celiac disease screening: Tests for antibodies associated with gluten intolerance.
    - Inflammatory markers: Tests such as C-reactive protein (CRP) or erythrocyte sedimentation rate (ESR) may be conducted to assess for signs of inflammation.
    - Thyroid function tests: Evaluate thyroid hormone levels, as thyroid disorders can contribute to gastrointestinal symptoms.
2. Stool Tests: Stool samples may be collected to check for:
    - Presence of blood: Helps rule out gastrointestinal bleeding.
    - Parasites or infections: Detects bacterial, viral, or parasitic infections.
    - Calprotectin or fecal lactoferrin: Measures levels of these markers to assess for inflammation in the digestive tract.
3. Imaging Tests:

- Colonoscopy: Involves inserting a flexible tube with a camera into the colon to visualize the entire colon and rectum. It helps evaluate for abnormalities, inflammation, or other gastrointestinal conditions.
  - Flexible sigmoidoscopy: Similar to colonoscopy, but examines only the lower part of the colon.
  - Abdominal ultrasound: Uses sound waves to create images of the abdominal organs, helping detect abnormalities or structural issues.
4. Hydrogen Breath Test: This test evaluates for certain types of carbohydrate malabsorption or intolerances, such as lactose intolerance or small intestinal bacterial overgrowth (SIBO).
5. Elimination Diets: A healthcare provider may recommend eliminating specific food groups, such as gluten or lactose, from your diet to assess if they are contributing to your symptoms. Gradual reintroduction of these foods can help identify any trigger foods.
6. Psychological Assessments: In some cases, healthcare providers may recommend psychological assessments, such as questionnaires or interviews, to evaluate the impact of stress, anxiety, or mood disorders on symptoms.

It's important to discuss these tests and evaluations with your healthcare provider, as they will determine which ones are most appropriate based on your symptoms, medical history, and clinical judgment. Remember, the diagnostic process for IBS involves a comprehensive evaluation, ruling out other conditions, and consideration of symptom patterns and medical history to make an accurate diagnosis.

IMPORTANCE OF CONSULTING A HEALTHCARE PROFESSIONAL

Consulting a healthcare professional is crucial when experiencing symptoms suggestive of Irritable Bowel Syndrome (IBS) or any other medical condition. Here are some reasons why it's important to seek medical advice:

1. Accurate Diagnosis: A healthcare professional can properly evaluate your symptoms, medical history, and conduct necessary tests to make an accurate diagnosis. This is important because IBS shares symptoms with other gastrointestinal disorders, and ruling out other conditions is essential for effective management.
2. Rule Out Other Conditions: Many gastrointestinal disorders have similar symptoms to IBS, but require different treatments. By consulting a healthcare professional, other potential causes of your symptoms can be investigated and ruled out. This ensures you receive appropriate care for your specific condition.
3. Individualized Treatment: Healthcare professionals can provide personalized treatment plans based on your symptoms, medical history, and diagnostic results. They can guide you in implementing lifestyle changes, dietary modifications, stress management techniques, and prescribe medications if needed. Tailored treatment helps manage symptoms effectively.
4. Monitoring and Follow-up: Regular consultations with a healthcare professional allow for monitoring of symptoms, treatment effectiveness, and adjustments if necessary. Follow-up appointments help ensure ongoing management of your condition and address any concerns or new symptoms that may arise.

5. Emotional Support: Living with a chronic condition like IBS can have an emotional impact. Healthcare professionals can offer emotional support, guidance, and provide resources to help you cope with the challenges associated with your condition. They can also address any psychological factors that may be contributing to your symptoms.

6. Prevention and Early Detection: Regular consultations with a healthcare professional can contribute to preventive care and early detection of any complications or additional health issues related to IBS or its management. It allows for proactive measures and timely interventions.

7. Education and Empowerment: Healthcare professionals can educate you about your condition, explain the nature of IBS, its triggers, and strategies for symptom management. This knowledge empowers you to make informed decisions and actively participate in your own healthcare.

Remember, healthcare professionals are trained to diagnose, manage, and support individuals with gastrointestinal disorders like IBS. They play a crucial role in guiding you through the diagnostic process, providing appropriate treatment, and improving your overall well-being. If you suspect you may have IBS or are experiencing persistent gastrointestinal symptoms, it is recommended to consult with a healthcare professional.

TYPES OF IBS

Irritable Bowel Syndrome (IBS) is classified into different types based on the predominant bowel habits and stool consistency experienced by individuals. The main types of IBS are as follows:

1. IBS with Constipation (IBS-C): This subtype of IBS is characterized by constipation as the predominant symptom. People with IBS-C typically have infrequent bowel movements, typically fewer than three bowel movements per week. They may experience difficulty passing stools and a sense of incomplete evacuation. Stools are often hard, lumpy, or pellet-like. Abdominal pain or discomfort may accompany constipation.
2. IBS with Diarrhea (IBS-D): IBS-D is characterized by diarrhea as the predominant symptom. Individuals with IBS-D experience frequent episodes of loose or watery stools. They often have an urgent need to have a bowel movement and may have difficulty controlling bowel movements. Abdominal pain or discomfort is commonly present and may be relieved after a bowel movement.
3. Mixed IBS (IBS-M): Mixed IBS, also known as IBS with Alternating Bowel Habits (IBS-A), is characterized by both constipation and diarrhea, with alternating episodes. People with IBS-M may have periods of constipation, where they experience infrequent bowel movements and difficulty passing stools. This is followed by episodes of diarrhea, with frequent loose or watery stools. The shift between constipation and diarrhea can vary in duration and frequency.
4. Unsubtyped IBS (IBS-U): Unsubtyped IBS refers to individuals who do not clearly fit into the categories of IBS-C or IBS-D. Their symptoms may not consistently align with

the predominant features of constipation or diarrhea. They may experience a mix of symptoms or have an unpredictable pattern of bowel habits.

It's important to note that individuals with IBS may also experience common symptoms that are not specific to a particular subtype. These symptoms can include abdominal pain or discomfort, bloating, excessive gas, and a sense of incomplete evacuation after a bowel movement. The severity and frequency of these symptoms can vary among individuals.

Understanding the subtype of IBS can provide some insight into the predominant bowel habits and guide initial treatment approaches. However, treatment plans for IBS are often individualized, focusing on symptom management and addressing underlying triggers, regardless of the subtype. It is advisable to consult with a healthcare professional to determine the most appropriate management plan based on your specific symptoms and needs.

EXPLORING THE DIFFERENT SUBTYPES OF IBS (IBS-C, IBS-D, IBS-M)

Let's explore the different subtypes of Irritable Bowel Syndrome (IBS) in more detail:

1. IBS with Constipation (IBS-C):
    - Predominant Symptoms: Constipation is the main feature of IBS-C. Individuals with this subtype typically have infrequent bowel movements, often less than three times per week.
    - Stool Characteristics: Stools tend to be hard, lumpy, or pellet-like, and individuals may experience difficulty passing them. They may also have a feeling of incomplete evacuation.
    - Abdominal Symptoms: Abdominal pain or discomfort is commonly present and may be relieved after a bowel movement.
    - Bloating and Gas: Individuals with IBS-C may also experience bloating and increased gas production.
2. IBS with Diarrhea (IBS-D):
    - Predominant Symptoms: Diarrhea is the primary symptom of IBS-D. People with this subtype experience frequent episodes of loose or watery stools.
    - Urgency and Bowel Control: There is often an urgent need to have a bowel movement, and individuals may struggle to control bowel movements, leading to occasional fecal incontinence.
    - Abdominal Symptoms: Abdominal pain or discomfort is commonly present, and it may be relieved after a bowel movement.

- o Bloating and Gas: Bloating and increased gas production may also occur in individuals with IBS-D.
3. Mixed IBS (IBS-M) or IBS with Alternating Bowel Habits (IBS-A):
   - o Predominant Symptoms: IBS-M is characterized by both constipation and diarrhea, with alternating episodes. Individuals may experience periods of constipation followed by episodes of diarrhea, or vice versa.
   - o Shifting Bowel Habits: The shift between constipation and diarrhea can vary in duration and frequency. Some individuals may notice a pattern of alternating symptoms over weeks or months.
   - o Abdominal Symptoms: Abdominal pain or discomfort is common and may be present regardless of the predominant bowel habit.
   - o Bloating and Gas: Bloating and excessive gas can occur in individuals with IBS-M.
4. Unsubtyped IBS (IBS-U):
   - o Characteristics: Unsubtyped IBS refers to individuals who do not fit clearly into the categories of IBS-C or IBS-D. Their symptoms may not consistently align with the predominant features of constipation or diarrhea, or they may experience a mix of symptoms without a predictable pattern.
   - o Variable Symptoms: Individuals with IBS-U may have a combination of constipation and diarrhea, but without a clear predominance of one over the other. Their bowel habits may fluctuate, and there may be variability in stool consistency.
   - o Abdominal Symptoms: Abdominal pain or discomfort is common in unsubtyped IBS, and it may not necessarily correlate with bowel movements.

- Bloating and Gas: Bloating and increased gas production can be experienced by individuals with unsubtyped IBS.

It's important to note that while the subtypes of IBS help to categorize predominant symptoms, many individuals with IBS may experience a mix of symptoms or transition between subtypes over time. Some individuals may even shift from one subtype to another.

The subtypes of IBS serve as a general framework to understand symptom patterns, but the focus of treatment is usually on managing individual symptoms and improving overall quality of life. Treatment approaches for IBS may include lifestyle modifications, dietary changes, stress management techniques, medications, and therapies tailored to the specific needs of the individual.

Remember, consulting with a healthcare professional is essential to receive an accurate diagnosis and develop an appropriate treatment plan based on your unique symptoms, medical history, and individual circumstances. They can help guide you in managing your symptoms effectively and improving your overall well-being.

It's important to note that individuals with IBS can experience additional symptoms such as abdominal bloating, increased gas, a feeling of incomplete evacuation, and mucus in the stool, regardless of the subtype.

While understanding the subtype can provide some guidance for treatment approaches, it's essential to remember that IBS is a complex condition and symptoms can overlap among subtypes. Treatment plans for IBS often focus on managing symptoms and addressing underlying triggers, irrespective of the subtype.

Consulting with a healthcare professional is crucial to receive an accurate diagnosis and develop an individualized treatment plan based on your specific symptoms and needs.

UNDERSTANDING THE UNIQUE CHALLENGES AND SYMPTOM PATTERNS OF EACH SUBTYPE

Certainly! Understanding the unique challenges and symptom patterns of each subtype of Irritable Bowel Syndrome (IBS) can provide insight into the specific experiences individuals may have. Here's a closer look at the challenges and symptom patterns associated with each subtype:

1. IBS with Constipation (IBS-C):
   - Challenges: The main challenge for individuals with IBS-C is the difficulty in passing stools and infrequent bowel movements. This can lead to discomfort, bloating, and a sense of incomplete evacuation.
   - Symptom Patterns: Symptom patterns in IBS-C often involve periods of constipation with hard, lumpy stools. Abdominal pain or discomfort is commonly experienced and may improve after a bowel movement.
2. IBS with Diarrhea (IBS-D):
   - Challenges: Individuals with IBS-D face challenges related to frequent and loose bowel movements, along with urgency and difficulty in controlling bowel movements. This can lead to anxiety and disrupt daily activities.
   - Symptom Patterns: The predominant symptom pattern in IBS-D is characterized by episodes of diarrhea, urgency to have a bowel movement, and abdominal pain or discomfort that may improve after a bowel movement.

3. Mixed IBS (IBS-M):
   - o Challenges: One of the key challenges for individuals with IBS-M is the unpredictable shifts between constipation and diarrhea. This can make it difficult to plan daily activities and may cause discomfort and frustration.
   - o Symptom Patterns: Symptom patterns in IBS-M involve alternating episodes of constipation and diarrhea. Individuals may experience periods of infrequent bowel movements followed by episodes of loose stools. Abdominal pain or discomfort can be present throughout these episodes.
4. Unsubtyped IBS (IBS-U):
   - o Challenges: The challenge for individuals with unsubtyped IBS lies in the unpredictable and variable nature of their symptoms. It may be challenging to identify specific triggers or patterns, making symptom management more complex.
   - o Symptom Patterns: In unsubtyped IBS, individuals may experience a mix of symptoms, with no clear predominance of constipation or diarrhea. They may have variable stool consistency and frequency, along with abdominal pain or discomfort and bloating.

It's important to note that these challenges and symptom patterns are generalizations, and individuals with IBS may experience unique variations or combinations of symptoms. Symptoms can also vary in severity and frequency over time.

Understanding the challenges and symptom patterns specific to each subtype can help healthcare professionals tailor treatment approaches and management strategies to address individual needs. Working closely with a healthcare professional can provide personalized guidance and support in navigating these challenges and finding effective symptom management strategies.

TRIGGERS AND LIFESTYLE FACTORS

Triggers and lifestyle factors play a significant role in the management of Irritable Bowel Syndrome (IBS). Identifying and understanding these triggers can help individuals with IBS make informed choices to minimize symptom flare-ups and improve their quality of life. Here are some common triggers and lifestyle factors to consider:

1. Diet:
    - Trigger Foods: Certain foods can trigger or worsen IBS symptoms. These may vary from person to person, but common triggers include fatty or fried foods, spicy foods, caffeine, alcohol, carbonated beverages, artificial sweeteners, high-fiber foods, and foods high in FODMAPs (fermentable carbohydrates).
    - Dietary Modifications: Keeping a food diary and eliminating or reducing potential trigger foods can help identify individual triggers. Working with a registered dietitian experienced in managing IBS can provide guidance on a suitable diet plan, such as the low FODMAP diet or other personalized approaches.
2. Stress and Emotional Well-being:
    - Stress Management: Stress and emotional factors can exacerbate IBS symptoms. Finding effective stress management techniques, such as relaxation exercises, meditation, deep breathing, yoga, or counseling, can help reduce symptom severity.
    - Emotional Support: Seeking emotional support from friends, family, or support groups can provide coping strategies and help reduce stress levels.

3. Exercise and Physical Activity:
    o Regular Exercise: Engaging in regular physical activity, such as walking, jogging, or yoga, can help regulate bowel movements, improve overall well-being, and reduce stress levels.
    o Individual Tolerance: Individuals with IBS may have different exercise tolerances, so finding an activity that suits their comfort level and doesn't trigger symptoms is important.
4. Sleep:
    o Prioritizing Quality Sleep: Adequate and restful sleep is crucial for managing IBS symptoms. Establishing a regular sleep routine, creating a comfortable sleep environment, and practicing good sleep hygiene can improve sleep quality and potentially reduce symptom severity.
5. Medication and Supplements:
    o Prescription Medications: Depending on symptom severity, healthcare professionals may prescribe medications to manage specific symptoms, such as antispasmodics for abdominal pain or discomfort, laxatives for constipation, or medications to regulate bowel movements.
    o Probiotics: Some individuals find relief from IBS symptoms by taking probiotic supplements, which may help promote a healthy gut microbiota balance. However, the specific strains and effectiveness vary, so it's best to consult with a healthcare professional before starting any supplements.
6. Hydration:
    o Maintaining Adequate Hydration: Drinking sufficient water throughout the day can help promote regular bowel movements and prevent constipation.

It's important for individuals with IBS to identify their personal triggers and adopt a holistic approach to managing their condition. This includes implementing lifestyle modifications, developing coping strategies for stress, and working closely with healthcare professionals to develop an individualized treatment plan.

IDENTIFYING TRIGGERS THAT WORSEN IBS SYMPTOMS (E.G., CERTAIN FOODS, STRESS)

Identifying triggers that worsen Irritable Bowel Syndrome (IBS) symptoms is a key step in managing the condition effectively. Triggers can vary from person to person, but here are some common triggers known to exacerbate IBS symptoms:

1. Specific Foods:
   - Fatty or Fried Foods: High-fat foods can stimulate contractions in the intestines, leading to diarrhea or abdominal discomfort in some individuals.
   - Spicy Foods: Spices and spicy foods may irritate the digestive tract and trigger symptoms such as abdominal pain or diarrhea.
   - Caffeine: Caffeinated beverages like coffee, tea, and certain sodas can stimulate the intestines and worsen diarrhea in some individuals.
   - Alcohol: Alcoholic beverages can act as gut irritants and trigger symptoms such as diarrhea, abdominal pain, or bloating.
   - Carbonated Beverages: The carbonation in sodas or fizzy drinks can cause gas and bloating in some individuals.
   - Artificial Sweeteners: Some artificial sweeteners, such as sorbitol, mannitol, or xylitol, may have a laxative effect and worsen diarrhea.
   - High-Fiber Foods: While fiber is generally beneficial for digestion, some high-fiber foods like beans, lentils, and certain fruits and vegetables can cause gas, bloating, or changes in bowel movements in individuals with IBS.
2. Emotional Factors and Stress:

- o Stress and Anxiety: Emotional stress, anxiety, and strong emotions can trigger or worsen IBS symptoms. The gut-brain connection plays a significant role in IBS, and stress can lead to increased sensitivity and abnormal functioning of the digestive system.
- o Psychological Factors: Depression, anxiety disorders, and other psychological conditions can influence IBS symptoms. Psychological support and stress management techniques can be helpful in managing these triggers.

3. Hormonal Changes:
- o Menstrual Cycle: Some individuals with IBS may notice that their symptoms worsen during certain phases of the menstrual cycle due to hormonal fluctuations.

4. Eating Habits:
- o Irregular Meal Times: Skipping meals or irregular eating patterns can disrupt the digestive system and trigger symptoms.
- o Overeating or Large Meals: Consuming large meals can overload the digestive system and lead to discomfort, bloating, or changes in bowel movements.

5. Medications and Supplements:
- o Certain medications or supplements, such as antibiotics, nonsteroidal anti-inflammatory drugs (NSAIDs), or magnesium supplements, may worsen IBS symptoms in some individuals. It's important to discuss with a healthcare professional about the potential impact of medications on IBS symptoms.

6. Environmental Factors:
- o Changes in Routine: Traveling, changes in daily routine, or disruptions in sleep patterns can

contribute to stress and trigger symptoms in individuals with IBS.

It's important for individuals with IBS to keep a symptom diary, noting the foods they eat, stress levels, and any other potential triggers. This can help identify patterns and specific triggers unique to their condition. Working with a healthcare professional, such as a registered dietitian experienced in managing IBS, can provide further guidance in identifying and managing specific triggers.

DISCUSSING LIFESTYLE FACTORS THAT CAN AFFECT IBS (E.G., DIET, EXERCISE, SLEEP)

Lifestyle factors play a significant role in managing Irritable Bowel Syndrome (IBS) and can have a direct impact on symptom severity and overall well-being. Here are some key lifestyle factors that can affect IBS:

1. Diet:
   - Dietary Modifications: Making specific changes to your diet can help manage IBS symptoms. Some general dietary guidelines include:
     - Eating Regularly: Establishing regular meal times and avoiding skipping meals can help maintain regular bowel function.
     - Balanced Fiber Intake: Consuming a balanced amount of dietary fiber can help regulate bowel movements. Some individuals with IBS may find relief by adjusting the type or amount of fiber in their diet. For example, increasing soluble fiber and reducing insoluble fiber may be beneficial.
     - Low-FODMAP Diet: Following a low-FODMAP diet may help alleviate symptoms for some individuals. FODMAPs are fermentable carbohydrates that can trigger symptoms in certain people. It involves temporarily eliminating high-FODMAP foods and gradually reintroducing them to identify individual triggers.
     - Identifying Trigger Foods: Keeping a food diary can help identify specific foods that

worsen your symptoms. Common triggers include spicy foods, fatty or fried foods, caffeine, alcohol, carbonated beverages, artificial sweeteners, and high-fat or high-fiber foods.

2. Exercise and Physical Activity:
    o Regular Exercise: Engaging in regular physical activity has been shown to have a positive impact on IBS symptoms. Exercise helps regulate bowel movements, reduce stress, and improve overall well-being. Activities such as walking, jogging, yoga, or cycling can be beneficial. It's important to find exercises that suit your individual tolerance and preferences.
    o Timing of Exercise: For some individuals, exercising before meals or allowing sufficient time for digestion after a meal can help minimize symptoms.
3. Stress Management:
    o Stress Reduction Techniques: Stress and anxiety can trigger or exacerbate IBS symptoms. Employing stress reduction techniques can be beneficial, such as deep breathing exercises, meditation, yoga, mindfulness practices, or engaging in hobbies and activities that promote relaxation.
    o Relaxation Techniques: Practicing relaxation techniques, such as progressive muscle relaxation or guided imagery, can help manage stress and promote a sense of well-being.
4. Sleep:
    o Consistent Sleep Routine: Maintaining a regular sleep schedule and prioritizing adequate sleep is important for managing IBS symptoms. Establishing a calming bedtime routine and creating a sleep-

friendly environment can promote better sleep quality.
   - o   Good Sleep Hygiene: Practicing good sleep hygiene, such as avoiding stimulating activities before bed, limiting exposure to electronic devices, and ensuring a comfortable sleep environment, can contribute to better sleep.
5. Hydration:
   - o   Sufficient Water Intake: Staying adequately hydrated is important for overall digestive health. Drinking enough water can help promote regular bowel movements and prevent constipation.
6. Smoking and Alcohol:
   - o   Smoking Cessation: Smoking has been linked to increased IBS symptoms. Quitting smoking can have a positive impact on both general health and IBS symptoms.
   - o   Alcohol Moderation: Excessive alcohol consumption can trigger or worsen symptoms for some individuals. Moderation or avoiding alcohol altogether may be beneficial.

It's important to note that lifestyle factors may affect individuals with IBS differently. It can be helpful to work with healthcare professionals, such as registered dietitians and therapists, who specialize in IBS management to develop a personalized approach tailored to your specific needs and triggers. Additionally, gradually implementing lifestyle changes and monitoring their effects on symptoms can help identify what works best for you.

MANAGING DIET AND NUTRITION

Managing diet and nutrition is an essential aspect of managing Irritable Bowel Syndrome (IBS) symptoms. Making specific dietary modifications can help reduce symptom severity and improve overall well-being. Here are some strategies for managing diet and nutrition in IBS:

1. Keep a Food Diary: Keeping a food diary can help identify trigger foods and patterns between your diet and symptoms. Record what you eat, when you eat it, and any symptoms that occur. This information can help pinpoint specific foods or ingredients that worsen your symptoms.
2. Low-FODMAP Diet: The low-FODMAP diet is an evidence-based approach that can help manage IBS symptoms for some individuals. FODMAPs are fermentable carbohydrates that can trigger digestive symptoms in susceptible individuals. The low-FODMAP diet involves eliminating high-FODMAP foods for a period of time and gradually reintroducing them to identify individual triggers. It is recommended to work with a registered dietitian experienced in the low-FODMAP diet to ensure proper guidance and nutrition.
3. Fiber Intake:
   o Soluble Fiber: Increasing soluble fiber intake can help regulate bowel movements and alleviate constipation. Good sources of soluble fiber include oats, barley, psyllium husk, flaxseeds, and certain fruits and vegetables like bananas, berries, and carrots.
   o Insoluble Fiber: Some individuals with IBS may be sensitive to high amounts of insoluble fiber. It may be helpful to limit or moderate intake from sources

such as bran, whole grains, and certain vegetables and fruits like cabbage, broccoli, and citrus fruits.

4. Small, Frequent Meals: Consuming smaller, more frequent meals instead of large meals can help prevent overloading the digestive system, which may contribute to symptoms.
5. Hydration: Drinking adequate water throughout the day helps maintain hydration and supports regular bowel movements. Aim to drink enough water based on your individual needs and activity level.
6. Probiotics: Probiotics are beneficial bacteria that can help improve gut health. Some studies suggest that certain probiotic strains may alleviate IBS symptoms. Talk to your healthcare provider about incorporating probiotics into your management plan.
7. Reduce Trigger Foods:
    o Identify Trigger Foods: Be aware of specific foods that consistently trigger your symptoms and consider reducing or eliminating them from your diet. Common triggers include fatty or fried foods, spicy foods, caffeine, alcohol, carbonated beverages, artificial sweeteners, and high-FODMAP foods.
    o Individual Tolerance: Each person with IBS may have unique trigger foods, so it's important to identify your personal triggers through trial and error.
8. Meal Planning and Preparation: Planning and preparing meals in advance can help ensure you have suitable options available and avoid relying on trigger foods or unhealthy choices when symptoms arise.
9. Consult with a Registered Dietitian: Working with a registered dietitian experienced in managing IBS can provide personalized guidance and support. They can help

develop a tailored diet plan, ensure nutritional adequacy, and assist in identifying trigger foods.

Remember, dietary management in IBS is highly individualized. What works for one person may not work for another. It's essential to consult with healthcare professionals, such as registered dietitians or gastroenterologists, who can provide personalized advice and help you navigate your specific dietary needs and goals.

OVERVIEW OF DIETARY STRATEGIES FOR IBS MANAGEMENT (E.G., LOW FODMAP DIET)

Managing irritable bowel syndrome (IBS) can be challenging, but dietary tactics can play a significant role in alleviating symptoms and improving overall well-being. One popular approach is the low FODMAP diet, which aims to reduce the intake of certain fermentable carbohydrates that can trigger IBS symptoms. Here are some dietary tactics, including the low FODMAP diet, that can be helpful for managing IBS:

Low FODMAP Diet: The low FODMAP diet involves avoiding or limiting foods high in fermentable carbohydrates such as lactose, fructose, fructans, galactans, and polyols. These carbohydrates can ferment in the gut, leading to symptoms like bloating, gas, abdominal pain, and diarrhea. Working with a registered dietitian experienced in the low FODMAP diet is recommended to ensure proper guidance and long-term management.

Identify Trigger Foods: Keep a food diary to track your symptoms and identify potential trigger foods. Common triggers can vary from person to person but may include spicy foods, fatty foods, caffeine, alcohol, and artificial sweeteners. By identifying and avoiding these trigger foods, you may experience a reduction in symptoms.

Fiber Management: Some individuals with IBS find relief by adjusting their fiber intake. Soluble fiber can help regulate bowel movements and alleviate constipation, while insoluble fiber may worsen symptoms in some cases. Experimenting with different fiber sources and adjusting the amount consumed can help determine what works best for your body.

Mindful Eating: Practicing mindful eating techniques can contribute to better digestion and symptom management. Slow down while eating, chew your food thoroughly, and pay attention to your body's hunger and fullness cues. Avoiding large meals and eating smaller, more frequent meals throughout the day may also help manage symptoms.

Stay Hydrated: Drinking plenty of water and staying hydrated can promote regular bowel movements and prevent constipation, which is a common symptom of IBS. Aim for at least 8 cups of water per day, but individual needs may vary.

Probiotics: Probiotics are beneficial bacteria that can help balance the gut microbiome and potentially alleviate IBS symptoms. Incorporating probiotic-rich foods like yogurt, kefir, sauerkraut, and kimchi into your diet or taking a probiotic supplement may be worth considering. However, consult with a healthcare professional to determine the most suitable probiotic strain and dosage for your specific needs.

Stress Management: Stress and anxiety can exacerbate IBS symptoms. Incorporating stress management techniques such as meditation, deep breathing exercises, regular exercise, and engaging in activities that promote relaxation can contribute to symptom relief.

Remember, it is crucial to consult with a healthcare professional or a registered dietitian who specializes in gastrointestinal disorders before making significant dietary changes. They can provide personalized advice and guidance based on your specific needs and medical history.

FOODS TO AVOID AND FOODS THAT MAY ALLEVIATE SYMPTOMS

When managing irritable bowel syndrome (IBS), it's important to identify and avoid trigger foods that can worsen symptoms. While trigger foods can vary from person to person, here are some commonly known foods to avoid if you have IBS:

High-FODMAP Foods: Fermentable carbohydrates known as FODMAPs (Fermentable Oligosaccharides, Disaccharides, Monosaccharides, and Polyols) can trigger IBS symptoms. Examples include:

Fructans: Found in wheat, rye, onions, garlic, and some fruits and vegetables.

Lactose: Found in dairy products like milk, cheese, and yogurt.

Fructose: Found in fruits like apples, pears, and honey.

Polyols: Found in sugar alcohols like sorbitol, mannitol, xylitol, and some fruits and vegetables like avocados and mushrooms.

Gas-Producing Foods: Certain foods can cause excessive gas production and bloating in individuals with IBS. Examples include beans, lentils, carbonated beverages, cruciferous vegetables (broccoli, cauliflower, cabbage), and onions.

Spicy and Acidic Foods: Spicy foods, hot sauces, and acidic foods like citrus fruits, tomatoes, and vinegar can be problematic for some individuals with IBS.

Caffeine and Alcohol: Both caffeine and alcohol can stimulate the digestive system and worsen IBS symptoms. It's advisable to limit or avoid coffee, tea, energy drinks, and alcoholic beverages.

While it's important to avoid trigger foods, some foods may provide relief or alleviate symptoms for individuals with IBS. These foods include:

Low-FODMAP Foods: Many low-FODMAP foods are well-tolerated and can be included in an IBS-friendly diet. Examples include rice, oats, quinoa, lean proteins (chicken, fish, tofu), certain fruits (e.g., bananas, grapes), and select vegetables (e.g., spinach, carrots, zucchini).

Soluble Fiber-Rich Foods: Soluble fiber can help regulate bowel movements and ease symptoms of constipation. Foods like oatmeal, psyllium husk, chia seeds, and flaxseeds are good sources of soluble fiber.

Peppermint: Peppermint has been shown to have a relaxing effect on the muscles of the gastrointestinal tract and may help relieve IBS symptoms. Peppermint tea or peppermint oil capsules may be beneficial for some individuals.

Ginger: Ginger has natural anti-inflammatory properties and can help soothe the digestive system. Consuming ginger tea or adding fresh ginger to meals may offer relief from IBS symptoms.

Probiotic Foods: Probiotic-rich foods like yogurt, kefir, sauerkraut, and kimchi contain beneficial bacteria that may help promote a healthy gut microbiome and improve IBS symptoms for some individuals.

Remember, it's essential to listen to your body and pay attention to how different foods affect your symptoms. Keep in mind that individual tolerances can vary, so it's best to work with a healthcare professional or registered dietitian who specializes in IBS to develop a personalized dietary plan that suits your specific needs.

MEAL PLANNING TIPS AND RECIPE SUGGESTIONS

Meal planning is an effective strategy for managing IBS symptoms and ensuring a well-balanced diet. Here are some tips and recipe suggestions to help you with your meal planning:

Focus on Low-FODMAP Ingredients: Since the low-FODMAP diet is commonly recommended for individuals with IBS, prioritize low-FODMAP ingredients in your meal planning. This includes foods like rice, quinoa, gluten-free oats, lean proteins (chicken, fish, tofu), low-FODMAP vegetables (carrots, zucchini, spinach), and low-FODMAP fruits (bananas, grapes, oranges).

Cook in Bulk: Prepare large batches of meals to save time and ensure you have IBS-friendly options readily available. This can include making a big pot of low-FODMAP soup, chili, or stir-fry that can be portioned and stored for later use.

Opt for Small, Frequent Meals: Eating smaller meals throughout the day rather than three large meals can help manage IBS symptoms. Plan for snacks or mini-meals that are easily digestible, such as a low-FODMAP yogurt with a handful of low-FODMAP granola or a small portion of grilled chicken with steamed low-FODMAP vegetables.

Incorporate Soluble Fiber: Include foods rich in soluble fiber to help regulate bowel movements. For example, you can add chia seeds to a smoothie, cook oatmeal with almond milk and top it with low-FODMAP fruits like strawberries, or create a salad with mixed greens and sliced carrots.

Experiment with Herbs and Spices: Instead of relying on high-FODMAP flavor enhancers like onions and garlic, explore the use of herbs and spices to add depth and flavor to your dishes. Try incorporating fresh basil, oregano, thyme, turmeric, or ginger to season your meals.

Mindful Cooking and Eating: Practice mindful cooking by paying attention to the ingredients you use and how they affect your symptoms. Similarly, practice mindful eating by savoring each bite, chewing thoroughly, and being present during mealtimes. This can help reduce stress and promote better digestion.

Seek Recipe Inspiration: There are many resources available that offer low-FODMAP recipes tailored for individuals with IBS. Look for cookbooks, online recipe databases, and reputable websites specializing in IBS-friendly cooking. Experiment with different recipes to keep your meals varied and enjoyable.

Here are a few recipe ideas to get you started:

Quinoa Salad with Grilled Chicken, Spinach, and Cherry Tomatoes

Low-FODMAP Stir-Fry with Tofu, Bell Peppers, and Bok Choy

Baked Salmon with Lemon and Dill, served with Roasted Carrots and Green Beans

Gluten-Free Oatmeal with Almond Milk, Blueberries, and a sprinkle of Chia Seeds

Low-FODMAP Chicken and Vegetable Soup seasoned with herbs like thyme and parsley

Remember, individual tolerances to certain ingredients may vary, so it's important to pay attention to your body's response to different foods. Consulting with a registered dietitian who specializes in IBS can provide personalized guidance and ensure your meal planning aligns with your specific dietary needs.

STRESS MANAGEMENT AND MENTAL HEALTH

Stress management and mental health are essential components of overall well-being. Here are some key points to consider when it comes to stress management and maintaining good mental health:

Recognize and Identify Stressors: Start by identifying the sources of stress in your life. These can be related to work, relationships, finances, health, or other aspects. By recognizing these stressors, you can begin to develop strategies to address them effectively.

Practice Self-Care: Taking care of yourself is crucial for managing stress and maintaining good mental health. This includes getting enough sleep, eating a balanced diet, engaging in regular physical activity, and allocating time for activities you enjoy.

Develop Healthy Coping Mechanisms: Find healthy ways to cope with stress, such as practicing relaxation techniques (deep breathing, meditation, yoga), engaging in hobbies or creative outlets, journaling, or seeking support from loved ones. Experiment with different strategies to determine what works best for you.

Prioritize Time for Rest and Relaxation: Allow yourself regular breaks and downtime to recharge. Engage in activities that help you relax and unwind, whether it's reading a book, taking a bath, listening to music, or spending time in nature.

Maintain a Supportive Social Network: Cultivate and nurture positive relationships with friends, family, and loved ones. Having a strong support system can provide emotional support, a listening ear, and a sense of belonging.

Seek Professional Help: If stress becomes overwhelming or starts to impact your daily life, consider reaching out to a mental health professional. They can provide guidance, support, and therapeutic interventions to help you manage stress effectively.

Practice Mindfulness: Mindfulness involves being fully present in the moment and non-judgmentally aware of your thoughts, feelings, and sensations. Regular mindfulness practice can help reduce stress, enhance self-awareness, and improve overall well-being.

Set Realistic Goals and Boundaries: Establishing realistic goals and setting boundaries can help manage stress and prevent overwhelm. Learn to say no when necessary, delegate tasks, and focus on what truly matters to you.

Engage in Physical Activity: Exercise is a powerful stress reliever and mood booster. Find physical activities that you enjoy and make them a regular part of your routine. Even small amounts of exercise can have significant benefits for mental health.

Limit Exposure to Stressors: Whenever possible, try to minimize your exposure to stressors that are within your control. This may involve setting boundaries with technology, managing your workload, or creating a peaceful environment at home.

Remember, everyone's experience with stress and mental health is unique. If you find yourself struggling, don't hesitate to reach out to professionals who can provide guidance and support. Taking proactive steps to manage stress and prioritize mental health is an investment in your overall well-being and quality of life.

PROVEN DIETRY THAT WORKED

Dietary strategies play a crucial role in managing Irritable Bowel Syndrome (IBS) symptoms. Here's an overview of some commonly used dietary approaches, including the Low FODMAP diet, for managing IBS:

1. Low FODMAP Diet:
    - Overview: The Low FODMAP diet is an evidence-based approach that aims to reduce the intake of fermentable carbohydrates known as FODMAPs (fermentable oligosaccharides, disaccharides, monosaccharides, and polyols).
    - FODMAPs and IBS: FODMAPs are poorly absorbed in the small intestine and can trigger symptoms such as abdominal pain, bloating, gas, and altered bowel habits in some individuals with IBS.
    - Phases of the Diet:
        - Elimination Phase: During this phase, high-FODMAP foods are eliminated from the diet for a specific period, typically 2 to 6 weeks. This phase aims to alleviate symptoms.
        - Reintroduction Phase: In this phase, FODMAP groups are systematically reintroduced one at a time to identify individual triggers and determine tolerance levels.
        - Personalization Phase: Once trigger foods are identified, an individualized long-term diet plan is developed, allowing for a balanced and varied diet while minimizing symptom triggers.

- o Working with a Dietitian: It is recommended to work with a registered dietitian experienced in the Low FODMAP diet to ensure proper guidance, support, and to maintain nutritional adequacy throughout the process.

2. Elimination of Trigger Foods:
   - o Identifying Triggers: Keeping a food diary can help identify specific trigger foods that worsen IBS symptoms. Common triggers include fatty or fried foods, spicy foods, caffeine, alcohol, carbonated beverages, artificial sweeteners, and high-fat or high-fiber foods.
   - o Individualized Approach: Trigger foods can vary from person to person, so it's important to identify your own specific triggers through trial and error.
   - o Collaboration with a Dietitian: Working with a registered dietitian can provide guidance in eliminating trigger foods while ensuring a balanced and nutritious diet.

3. Fiber Modifications:
   - o Soluble Fiber: Increasing intake of soluble fiber can help regulate bowel movements and alleviate constipation. Good sources include oats, barley, psyllium husk, flaxseeds, and certain fruits and vegetables.
   - o Moderating Insoluble Fiber: Some individuals with IBS may be sensitive to high amounts of insoluble fiber. Moderating intake from sources such as bran, whole grains, and certain vegetables and fruits can be helpful.

4. Adequate Hydration:
   - o Drinking enough water throughout the day helps maintain hydration and supports regular bowel

movements. Aim to drink adequate water based on your individual needs and activity level.

5. Individualized Approaches:
    o Each person with IBS may have unique dietary needs and triggers, so it's important to find an approach that works for you. Working with a registered dietitian can help develop an individualized diet plan tailored to your specific needs.

It's important to note that dietary management in IBS is highly individual, and what works for one person may not work for another. Consulting with healthcare professionals, such as registered dietitians or gastroenterologists, who specialize in IBS management is recommended to receive personalized guidance, support, and to ensure nutritional adequacy while managing your symptoms effectively.

THE IMPACT OF STRESS AND ANXIETY ON IBS SYMPTOMS

Stress and anxiety can have a significant impact on the symptoms of irritable bowel syndrome (IBS). Here's how stress and anxiety can influence IBS symptoms:

Gut-Brain Connection: The gut and the brain are closely connected through the gut-brain axis. Stress and anxiety can disrupt the balance of the gut-brain axis, leading to changes in gut motility, sensitivity, and function. This can trigger or worsen IBS symptoms.

Increased Sensitivity: Stress and anxiety can make the gastrointestinal tract more sensitive to normal digestive processes. This means that even mild changes in the gut, such as the presence of gas or normal muscle contractions, can be perceived as pain or discomfort in individuals with IBS.

Altered Gut Motility: Stress and anxiety can impact the normal movement of the digestive system, leading to changes in bowel habits. Some individuals may experience increased motility, resulting in diarrhea, while others may experience decreased motility, leading to constipation.

Enhanced Pain Perception: Stress and anxiety can lower the pain threshold, making individuals with IBS more sensitive to pain. This can intensify the severity of abdominal pain or discomfort associated with IBS.

Increased Inflammation: Chronic stress and anxiety can contribute to low-grade inflammation in the body, including the gastrointestinal tract. Inflammation can further exacerbate IBS symptoms and contribute to overall gut dysfunction.

Changes in Gut Microbiota: Stress and anxiety can affect the composition and diversity of the gut microbiota, which plays a crucial role in gut health. Imbalances in the gut microbiota have been linked to IBS symptoms, and stress-related changes in the microbiota can potentially worsen symptoms.

It's important to note that while stress and anxiety can influence IBS symptoms, they do not cause IBS. IBS is a complex disorder with multiple factors involved, including genetic predisposition, gut dysregulation, and environmental factors.

Managing stress and anxiety is crucial for individuals with IBS to alleviate symptoms and improve quality of life. Here are some strategies that can help:

Stress Management Techniques: Practice stress-reduction techniques such as deep breathing exercises, meditation, mindfulness, yoga, or engaging in hobbies that promote relaxation. Find activities that help you unwind and release tension.

Regular Exercise: Engage in regular physical activity as it can help reduce stress and promote overall well-being. Choose activities that you enjoy and that suit your fitness level.

Cognitive Behavioral Therapy (CBT): CBT is a therapeutic approach that focuses on identifying and changing negative thought patterns and behaviors. It can be helpful in managing stress, anxiety, and coping with IBS symptoms.

Support System: Seek support from friends, family, or support groups. Sharing your experiences with others who understand can provide emotional support and coping strategies.

Prioritize Self-Care: Make self-care a priority. Take time for activities that bring you joy and relaxation. This can include hobbies, spending time in nature, reading, or practicing self-care rituals.

Seek Professional Help: If stress and anxiety become overwhelming, consider seeking help from a mental health professional. They can provide guidance, support, and interventions tailored to your specific needs.

By effectively managing stress and anxiety, individuals with IBS can potentially reduce the frequency and severity of symptoms, improving their overall well-being and quality of life.

STRESS REDUCTION TECHNIQUES (E.G., RELAXATION EXERCISES, MINDFULNESS)

Stress reduction techniques can be beneficial in managing the symptoms of Irritable Bowel Syndrome (IBS), as stress can exacerbate IBS symptoms. Here are some commonly used stress reduction techniques that may help:

1. Relaxation Exercises:
   - Deep Breathing: Deep breathing exercises can help activate the body's relaxation response. Take slow, deep breaths, inhaling through your nose and exhaling through your mouth.
   - Progressive Muscle Relaxation: This technique involves progressively tensing and then releasing different muscle groups in the body, promoting a sense of relaxation and reducing muscle tension.
   - Guided Imagery: Guided imagery involves using your imagination to visualize calm and peaceful scenes, such as a beach or a forest. Guided imagery recordings or apps can assist in the process.
2. Mindfulness and Meditation:
   - Mindfulness Meditation: Mindfulness involves focusing your attention on the present moment without judgment. It can help reduce stress and enhance overall well-being. Practices like body scan meditation or mindful breathing can be beneficial.
   - Meditation Apps: Utilize meditation apps, such as Headspace, Calm, or Insight Timer, which provide guided meditations and mindfulness exercises.
3. Yoga and Tai Chi:
   - Yoga: Yoga combines physical postures, breathing techniques, and meditation. It promotes relaxation,

flexibility, and stress reduction. Gentle forms of yoga, such as Hatha or Restorative Yoga, may be particularly beneficial for individuals with IBS.

- o Tai Chi: Tai Chi is a mind-body practice that involves slow, gentle movements and deep breathing. It can promote relaxation, improve body awareness, and reduce stress.

4. Exercise:

- o Regular Exercise: Engaging in regular physical activity, such as walking, jogging, swimming, or cycling, can help reduce stress levels and improve overall well-being. Find an exercise routine that suits your preferences and individual tolerance.

5. Journaling:

- o Stress Journaling: Keeping a journal can be a helpful way to identify and explore sources of stress and emotions related to your IBS symptoms. Writing down your thoughts and feelings can provide a sense of release and perspective.

6. Social Support:

- o Seek Support: Engage with friends, family, or support groups who can provide emotional support and understanding. Sharing experiences with others who have IBS can be helpful in coping with stress and managing symptoms.

7. Time Management and Self-Care:

- o Prioritize Self-Care: Engaging in activities that bring you joy and relaxation is essential for stress management. Dedicate time to hobbies, interests, and self-care practices that promote overall well-being.

- o Time Management: Managing your time effectively, setting realistic goals, and prioritizing tasks can help

reduce stress levels and create a sense of balance in
your daily life.

Remember, everyone responds differently to stress reduction
techniques, so it's important to find what works best for you.
Integrating these techniques into your daily routine and
maintaining consistency can enhance their effectiveness. If stress
levels or symptoms persist, consider seeking support from mental
health professionals who specialize in stress management
techniques or cognitive-behavioral therapy.

SEEKING SUPPORT AND THERAPY OPTIONS

Seeking support and therapy can be immensely beneficial for managing stress, anxiety, and the symptoms of conditions like IBS. Here are some therapy options and support avenues to consider:

Cognitive Behavioral Therapy (CBT): CBT is a widely used therapeutic approach that focuses on identifying and changing negative thought patterns and behaviors. It can help individuals develop effective coping strategies, challenge irrational beliefs, and manage stress and anxiety. CBT can be delivered in individual or group settings.

Psychodynamic Therapy: Psychodynamic therapy explores the underlying factors that contribute to stress, anxiety, and other psychological issues. It aims to increase self-awareness, understand patterns of behavior, and work through unresolved emotional conflicts. This therapy is typically conducted in one-on-one sessions.

Mindfulness-Based Stress Reduction (MBSR): MBSR combines mindfulness meditation, body awareness, and yoga to help individuals cultivate greater awareness and acceptance of the present moment. It can be beneficial for reducing stress, improving emotional well-being, and enhancing coping skills.

Support Groups: Joining a support group can provide a sense of community and understanding. Interacting with others who share similar experiences can offer emotional support, practical advice, and validation. Support groups may be in-person or online, and they can be specific to IBS or general mental health.

Online Counseling and Therapy Platforms: Online counseling and therapy platforms provide convenient access to licensed therapists through secure video or text-based sessions. These platforms offer a wide range of therapeutic approaches and allow you to receive support from the comfort of your own home.

Integrative Therapies: Various complementary and alternative therapies, such as acupuncture, hypnotherapy, and relaxation techniques, can be considered as part of a holistic approach to managing stress, anxiety, and IBS symptoms. These therapies can be used in conjunction with traditional therapy approaches.

Healthcare Professionals: Consult with healthcare professionals who specialize in IBS and mental health. Gastroenterologists, psychologists, psychiatrists, and registered dietitians can offer guidance, prescribe medications if necessary, and develop personalized treatment plans.

Remember, finding the right form of therapy and support is a personal journey. It's important to explore different options and find a therapist or support system that aligns with your needs and preferences. Seeking professional help can provide valuable tools, insights, and strategies to effectively manage stress, anxiety, and the impact they have on IBS symptoms.

MEDICATIONS AND MEDICAL TREATMENTS

Medications and medical treatments can be part of the management plan for Irritable Bowel Syndrome (IBS) when lifestyle modifications alone are insufficient in controlling symptoms. Here are some common medications and medical treatments used for IBS:

1. Over-the-Counter (OTC) Medications:
   - Antidiarrheal Medications: OTC medications, such as loperamide, can help alleviate diarrhea symptoms by slowing down bowel movements. They are generally used on an as-needed basis.
   - Fiber Supplements: For individuals with IBS-C, fiber supplements, such as psyllium husk or methylcellulose, can help increase stool bulk and promote regular bowel movements.
2. Prescription Medications:
   - Antispasmodic Medications: Prescription antispasmodics, such as dicyclomine or hyoscyamine, can help reduce abdominal pain and cramping by relaxing the muscles in the gastrointestinal tract.
   - Tricyclic Antidepressants (TCAs): Certain TCAs, such as amitriptyline or nortriptyline, in low doses, can help alleviate IBS symptoms, including abdominal pain, by affecting nerve signals in the gut.
   - Selective Serotonin Reuptake Inhibitors (SSRIs): SSRIs, such as fluoxetine or sertraline, may be prescribed for individuals with IBS to help manage abdominal pain and improve overall well-being.
   - Medications for Diarrhea-Predominant IBS (IBS-D): Prescription medications, such as alosetron or

rifaximin, may be used specifically for managing diarrhea symptoms in individuals with IBS-D. These medications are usually reserved for individuals with severe symptoms who haven't responded to other treatments.
- o Medications for Constipation-Predominant IBS (IBS-C): Prescription medications, such as lubiprostone or linaclotide, may be prescribed to help relieve constipation and improve bowel movements in individuals with IBS-C.

3. Psychological Therapies:
- o Cognitive-Behavioral Therapy (CBT): CBT is a form of therapy that focuses on identifying and modifying negative thoughts and behaviors related to IBS. It can help individuals develop coping strategies and manage stress, anxiety, and the impact of IBS on their daily life.
- o Gut-Directed Hypnotherapy: This specialized form of therapy uses relaxation and hypnosis techniques to help manage IBS symptoms, particularly abdominal pain and altered bowel habits.

4. Probiotics:
- o Probiotic Supplements: Probiotics are beneficial bacteria that can help improve gut health. Certain strains of probiotics have shown promise in alleviating IBS symptoms in some individuals. Probiotic supplements may be recommended, but the specific strains and effectiveness can vary, so it's important to consult with a healthcare professional before starting any supplements.

It's important to note that medication options and treatments may vary depending on the specific symptoms and subtype of IBS. The choice of medications or medical treatments should be made in consultation with a healthcare professional who can evaluate your symptoms, medical history, and individual needs. They can help determine the most appropriate treatment approach and monitor your response to medications.

OVERVIEW OF COMMON MEDICATIONS PRESCRIBED FOR IBS

Several medications may be prescribed to help manage the symptoms of irritable bowel syndrome (IBS). It's important to note that the choice of medication depends on the specific symptoms and needs of the individual. Here's an overview of common medications prescribed for IBS:

Antispasmodics: Antispasmodic medications help to relieve abdominal pain and cramping associated with IBS. They work by relaxing the muscles in the digestive tract. Examples of antispasmodics include hyoscine (scopolamine), dicyclomine, and peppermint oil capsules.

Fiber Supplements: Fiber supplements, such as psyllium husk or methylcellulose, may be recommended for individuals with IBS-C (constipation-predominant IBS). These supplements help add bulk to the stool and promote regular bowel movements.

Laxatives: Laxatives may be prescribed for individuals with IBS-C to help relieve constipation. Different types of laxatives, such as osmotic laxatives, stool softeners, or stimulant laxatives, may be used depending on the severity of constipation.

Probiotics: Probiotics are beneficial bacteria that can help restore the balance of gut flora and improve symptoms in some individuals with IBS. They may help alleviate bloating, gas, and irregular bowel movements. Different strains and formulations of probiotics are available, so it's important to choose one that is specifically targeted for IBS.

Antidepressants: Certain classes of antidepressant medications, such as tricyclic antidepressants (TCAs) or selective serotonin reuptake inhibitors (SSRIs), may be prescribed for individuals with IBS. These medications can help relieve pain, improve bowel habits, and manage anxiety or depression that often coexist with IBS.

Medications for Diarrhea Control: For individuals with IBS-D (diarrhea-predominant IBS), medications like loperamide or eluxadoline may be prescribed to help reduce diarrhea and improve stool consistency. These medications work by slowing down bowel movements.

It's important to consult with a healthcare professional, such as a gastroenterologist, to determine the most appropriate medication for your specific symptoms and medical history. They will consider factors such as the predominant symptoms (constipation, diarrhea, or mixed), overall health, and potential interactions with other medications.

It's worth noting that medications are often used in conjunction with lifestyle changes, dietary modifications (such as a low-FODMAP diet), and stress management techniques to provide comprehensive symptom relief and improve overall quality of life for individuals with IBS.

EXPLORING ALTERNATIVE THERAPIES (E.G., PROBIOTICS, HERBAL SUPPLEMENTS)

Alternative therapies are sometimes considered as complementary approaches to managing Irritable Bowel Syndrome (IBS) symptoms. While the evidence for their effectiveness varies, some individuals may find relief or improvement in symptoms with these therapies. Here are a few examples:

1. Probiotics:
    - Probiotic Supplements: Probiotics are live microorganisms that, when consumed in adequate amounts, can provide health benefits by promoting a healthy balance of gut bacteria. Some studies suggest that certain probiotic strains may help alleviate IBS symptoms, although results are mixed and vary among individuals. Examples of commonly studied probiotic strains for IBS include Bifidobacterium infantis, Lactobacillus acidophilus, and Saccharomyces boulardii. It's important to choose a reputable brand and consult with a healthcare professional before starting probiotic supplements.
2. Herbal Supplements:
    - Peppermint Oil: Peppermint oil, particularly enteric-coated capsules, may help reduce symptoms such as abdominal pain, bloating, and gas. It acts as an antispasmodic agent, relaxing the muscles of the gastrointestinal tract. However, it's important to note that peppermint oil may not be suitable for everyone, as it can cause heartburn or worsen symptoms in some individuals.

- o Other Herbal Supplements: Various herbal supplements, such as chamomile, fennel, ginger, and turmeric, have been used traditionally for digestive health and may provide symptom relief for some individuals. However, scientific evidence supporting their effectiveness for IBS is limited, and the safety and efficacy of herbal supplements can vary. It's important to consult with a healthcare professional before using herbal supplements, as they can interact with medications or have side effects.

3. Acupuncture:
   - o Acupuncture is an ancient Chinese therapy that involves inserting thin needles into specific points on the body. Some studies suggest that acupuncture may help reduce pain and improve overall well-being in individuals with IBS. However, more research is needed to establish its effectiveness and determine the appropriate treatment protocols.

4. Mind-Body Techniques:
   - o Relaxation Techniques: Relaxation exercises, such as deep breathing, progressive muscle relaxation, and guided imagery, can help reduce stress and alleviate IBS symptoms. They promote a state of relaxation and may positively impact overall well-being.
   - o Hypnotherapy: Gut-directed hypnotherapy is a specialized form of therapy that uses relaxation and hypnosis techniques to help manage IBS symptoms, particularly abdominal pain and altered bowel habits. It aims to modify the brain-gut interactions and has shown promising results in some studies.

It's important to note that while alternative therapies may be appealing, the scientific evidence supporting their effectiveness for IBS is often limited or mixed. Additionally, what works for one individual may not work for another. It's essential to consult with a healthcare professional before starting any alternative therapy to ensure safety and appropriateness for your specific situation. They can provide guidance, assess potential interactions or side effects, and help you make informed decisions regarding alternative therapies.

DISCUSSING THE POTENTIAL BENEFITS AND LIMITATIONS OF MEDICAL INTERVENTIONS

Medical interventions, such as medications, can provide relief and improve symptoms for individuals with irritable bowel syndrome (IBS). However, it's important to understand both the potential benefits and limitations associated with these interventions. Here's a discussion of their key aspects:

Benefits of Medical Interventions for IBS:

Symptom Relief: Medications can help alleviate specific symptoms of IBS, such as abdominal pain, cramping, diarrhea, constipation, and bloating. They can provide short-term relief and improve overall comfort.

Improved Quality of Life: By reducing the severity and frequency of symptoms, medical interventions can enhance the quality of life for individuals with IBS. They may experience fewer disruptions in daily activities and have better emotional well-being.

Targeted Approach: Medications can specifically target the predominant symptom of IBS, whether it's constipation, diarrhea, or pain. This allows for more personalized treatment and symptom management.

Complementary to Lifestyle Changes: Medical interventions can work in conjunction with lifestyle modifications, dietary adjustments (such as a low-FODMAP diet), and stress management techniques to provide comprehensive relief and support overall management of IBS.

Limitations of Medical Interventions for IBS:

Variable Effectiveness: Not all medications work equally well for everyone with IBS. Response to medications can vary depending on individual factors and the specific subtype of IBS. Some individuals may find significant relief, while others may experience minimal benefit or encounter side effects.

Side Effects: Like any medication, interventions for IBS can have potential side effects. These may include drowsiness, dry mouth, constipation, diarrhea, nausea, and others. It's important to discuss potential side effects with your healthcare provider and weigh them against the potential benefits.

Long-Term Management: Medical interventions generally focus on symptom relief rather than curing IBS. They may need to be taken continuously or intermittently to maintain symptom control. Long-term reliance on medication may not be preferable for some individuals.

Individual Variability: Each person with IBS is unique, and what works for one individual may not work for another. It may require trial and error to find the most effective medication and dosage for an individual's specific symptoms and needs.

Holistic Approach: While medications can provide relief, they may not address the underlying factors contributing to IBS, such as stress, anxiety, dietary triggers, or gut dysbiosis. A holistic approach that combines medical interventions with lifestyle modifications, stress management, and psychological support may be necessary for comprehensive management.

It's important to work closely with a healthcare professional, such as a gastroenterologist, to explore and understand the potential benefits and limitations of medical interventions for IBS. They can provide guidance, monitor your progress, and make adjustments to your treatment plan as needed.

LIFESTYLE ADJUSTMENTS FOR IBS

Lifestyle adjustments can play a significant role in managing Irritable Bowel Syndrome (IBS) symptoms. Here are some key lifestyle adjustments that may help:

1. Diet and Eating Habits:
    - Keep a Food Diary: Keeping a record of your food intake and symptoms can help identify trigger foods and patterns. This can guide you in making targeted dietary adjustments.
    - Balanced and Regular Meals: Establish regular meal times and aim for balanced meals that include a variety of nutrient-rich foods.
    - High-Fiber Foods: Gradually increase fiber intake from sources like whole grains, fruits, vegetables, and legumes, if tolerated. However, individuals with IBS may have varying tolerance to fiber, so it's important to find the right balance.
    - Fluid Intake: Drink adequate water throughout the day to maintain hydration and support regular bowel movements.
    - Limit Trigger Foods: Identify and reduce or eliminate foods that consistently trigger your symptoms. Common triggers include fatty or fried foods, spicy foods, caffeine, alcohol, carbonated beverages, artificial sweeteners, and high-fat or high-fiber foods.
2. Stress Management:
    - Relaxation Techniques: Practice relaxation exercises such as deep breathing, progressive muscle relaxation, and guided imagery to reduce stress levels and promote overall well-being.

- o Mindfulness and Meditation: Engage in mindfulness practices and meditation to cultivate present-moment awareness and reduce stress.
  - o Exercise: Regular physical activity, such as walking, jogging, yoga, or swimming, can help reduce stress and promote relaxation.
3. Sleep:
  - o Prioritize Sleep: Establish a regular sleep schedule and create a conducive sleep environment to ensure sufficient and restful sleep.
4. Regular Physical Activity:
  - o Engage in Regular Exercise: Regular physical activity helps regulate bowel movements, reduce stress, and improve overall well-being. Find activities that you enjoy and are suitable for your individual tolerance level.
5. Hydration:
  - o Drink Enough Water: Staying adequately hydrated promotes regular bowel movements and helps prevent constipation.
6. Smoking and Alcohol:
  - o Quit Smoking: If you smoke, consider quitting, as smoking can worsen symptoms and negatively impact overall health.
  - o Moderate Alcohol Intake: Limit alcohol consumption or avoid it altogether, as excessive alcohol intake can trigger or worsen IBS symptoms.
7. Support and Self-Care:
  - o Seek Support: Connect with support groups, friends, or family members who can provide emotional support and understanding.
  - o Self-Care Practices: Engage in self-care activities that promote relaxation, stress reduction, and overall well-being, such as hobbies, leisure

activities, or practices that bring you joy and relaxation.

Remember, lifestyle adjustments for managing IBS should be individualized. It may take time and experimentation to identify what works best for you. Working with healthcare professionals, such as registered dietitians, therapists, or gastroenterologists, can provide personalized guidance and support in implementing and maintaining lifestyle adjustments that suit your specific needs and preferences.

TIPS FOR MANAGING DAILY ROUTINES WITH IBS

Managing daily routines with irritable bowel syndrome (IBS) can be challenging, but with some adjustments and strategies, it's possible to minimize the impact of symptoms on your day-to-day life. Here are some tips to help manage your daily routines with IBS:

Establish a Routine: Establishing a regular routine for meals, sleep, and physical activity can help regulate your digestive system. Try to eat meals at consistent times, get enough sleep, and incorporate regular exercise into your daily routine.

Mindful Eating: Practice mindful eating by paying attention to your body's hunger and fullness cues. Eat slowly, chew your food thoroughly, and take breaks between bites. This can help prevent overeating and reduce the likelihood of triggering IBS symptoms.

Monitor Your Triggers: Keep a food and symptom diary to identify any specific triggers that worsen your symptoms. Common triggers include certain foods (e.g., high-FODMAP foods), stress, caffeine, alcohol, and artificial sweeteners. Once you identify your triggers, try to avoid or limit them as much as possible.

Plan Meals and Snacks: Plan your meals and snacks in advance to ensure you have access to suitable options throughout the day. Pack portable and easily digestible snacks, such as fruits, low-FODMAP granola bars, or rice cakes, when you're on the go. This helps prevent hunger-induced symptoms or the temptation to make less ideal food choices.

Stay Hydrated: Drink an adequate amount of water throughout the day to maintain hydration and promote healthy digestion. Avoid excessive consumption of carbonated beverages, as they can contribute to bloating and gas.

Stress Management: Develop effective stress management techniques that work for you. This can include activities such as deep breathing exercises, meditation, yoga, journaling, or engaging in hobbies that help you relax. Managing stress can have a positive impact on your IBS symptoms.

Bathroom Access: Ensure you have easy access to bathrooms when you're away from home. Familiarize yourself with the locations of restrooms in places you frequent, and plan your outings accordingly to reduce anxiety and discomfort.

Communication: If necessary, communicate your needs to trusted friends, family, or colleagues. Let them know about your condition and any specific requirements you may have. This can help alleviate stress or anxiety associated with social situations.

Seek Support: Connect with support groups or online communities where you can share experiences and learn from others with IBS. Having a support system can provide emotional support, practical advice, and a sense of understanding.

Consult a Healthcare Professional: Work closely with a healthcare professional, such as a gastroenterologist or registered dietitian, who specializes in IBS. They can provide personalized guidance, recommend dietary modifications, and suggest appropriate treatment options to help manage your symptoms.

Remember, everyone's experience with IBS is unique, so it may take some trial and error to find the strategies that work best for you. Be patient with yourself, prioritize self-care, and focus on finding a balance that supports your overall well-being while managing your IBS symptoms.

STRATEGIES FOR HANDLING SOCIAL SITUATIONS AND TRAVEL

Handling social situations and travel can pose challenges for individuals with Irritable Bowel Syndrome (IBS). Here are some strategies to help navigate these situations:

1. Social Situations:
   - Communication: Communicate your needs and concerns to trusted friends, family, or event organizers. Let them know about your condition and any dietary restrictions or accommodations you require.
   - Plan Ahead: If you're attending an event or gathering, inquire about the food options available. If possible, offer to bring a dish that aligns with your dietary needs to ensure there's something you can safely consume.
   - Mindful Eating: Practice mindful eating techniques, such as eating slowly, chewing thoroughly, and paying attention to your body's cues of fullness. This can help prevent overeating and minimize discomfort.
   - Limit Trigger Foods: Be mindful of trigger foods in social situations and opt for alternatives that are more compatible with your dietary needs. Choose foods that are less likely to trigger symptoms or bring your own snacks if necessary.
   - Stress Management: Use stress reduction techniques, such as deep breathing or visualization exercises, to manage stress and anxiety in social situations, as stress can exacerbate IBS symptoms.
2. Travel:

- Plan Ahead: Research and plan your travel arrangements, including access to restrooms, meal options, and potential triggers at your destination.
  - Pack Smart: Pack necessary medications, snacks, and any specific dietary items that you may need during your travels. Consider having a portable toilet kit or extra supplies on hand, such as toilet paper or wet wipes.
  - Stay Hydrated: Drink sufficient water throughout your journey to stay hydrated and support regular bowel movements.
  - Adjust Meal Choices: When dining out while traveling, choose simpler dishes that are less likely to contain trigger ingredients. Opt for grilled or baked options and request modifications or substitutions if needed.
  - Manage Stress: Travel can be stressful, so implement stress management techniques like deep breathing, mindfulness, or listening to calming music to help reduce stress levels.
  - Allow for Rest: Ensure you have ample rest periods during your travel to minimize fatigue and promote overall well-being.

3. Open Communication:
   - Inform Travel Companions: If you're traveling with others, inform them about your condition, triggers, and any specific needs. This helps create an understanding and supportive environment.
   - Request Accommodations: If needed, don't hesitate to request accommodations, such as access to restrooms or dietary modifications, from airlines, hotels, or other travel providers. Many are willing to accommodate special requests.

4. Flexibility and Self-Compassion:

- o Be Flexible: Recognize that unexpected situations can arise during social events or travel. Approach them with flexibility and adaptability, knowing that you may need to make adjustments to manage your symptoms effectively.
- o Practice Self-Compassion: Remember to be kind to yourself. Understand that managing IBS can be challenging, and occasional setbacks are normal. Focus on self-care and prioritize your well-being.

By planning ahead, communicating your needs, and employing strategies to manage stress and dietary choices, you can navigate social situations and travel with greater ease. Experiment with different approaches to find what works best for you, and remember to consult with healthcare professionals for personalized advice and guidance based on your specific condition and needs.

MAINTAINING A HEALTHY WORK-LIFE BALANCE

Maintaining a healthy work-life balance is crucial for overall well-being, including managing symptoms of conditions like Irritable Bowel Syndrome (IBS). Here are some strategies to help achieve and maintain a healthy work-life balance:

1. Prioritize Self-Care:
   - Set Boundaries: Establish clear boundaries between work and personal life. Define specific working hours and try to disconnect from work-related tasks outside of those hours.
   - Take Breaks: Take regular breaks during the workday to rest, stretch, and recharge. Incorporate short walks or relaxation exercises to reduce stress and improve focus.
   - Engage in Hobbies and Activities: Dedicate time to activities you enjoy outside of work, such as hobbies, exercise, reading, or spending time with loved ones. These activities help promote relaxation and bring balance to your life.
   - Practice Stress Management Techniques: Engage in stress reduction techniques, such as mindfulness, deep breathing, or meditation, to manage stress levels and promote overall well-being.
2. Time Management and Organization:
   - Prioritize Tasks: Identify the most important tasks and prioritize them based on deadlines and importance. This helps manage workload and reduces the risk of feeling overwhelmed.

- o Delegate: If possible, delegate tasks to others to lighten your workload and create more time for personal activities.
  - o Plan and Schedule: Use time management techniques, such as creating to-do lists or using digital calendars, to plan and schedule tasks, meetings, and personal activities. This helps ensure a balanced distribution of time and commitments.
  - o Avoid Overcommitment: Learn to say no to additional responsibilities or tasks that may overload your schedule. Focus on what truly aligns with your priorities and values.

3. Open Communication:
  - o Communicate Boundaries: Clearly communicate your work-life balance needs and boundaries to your supervisor, colleagues, and clients. This allows others to understand and respect your limits.
  - o Request Flexibility: If feasible, explore flexible work arrangements, such as flexible hours or remote work options, to accommodate your specific needs and promote work-life balance.

4. Disconnect from Work:
  - o Digital Detox: Take regular breaks from electronic devices, especially outside of work hours. Set aside dedicated time without checking work-related emails or messages to create space for personal activities and relaxation.
  - o Engage in Activities That Help You Unwind: Engage in activities that help you disconnect from work and unwind, such as exercise, reading, spending time in nature, or pursuing creative endeavors.

5. Seek Support:
  - o Build a Supportive Network: Cultivate relationships with colleagues, friends, and family who understand

and support your efforts to maintain a healthy work-life balance. Lean on them for support and encouragement.

- o Utilize Employee Assistance Programs (EAP): If available, take advantage of EAP resources that provide counseling, stress management tools, and support for work-life balance.

Remember, achieving work-life balance is an ongoing process that requires conscious effort and adjustment. It may vary depending on individual circumstances and priorities. Regularly reassess your balance, make necessary adjustments, and prioritize self-care to ensure long-term well-being.

COPING WITH FLARE-UPS AND SYMPTOM MANAGEMENT

Coping with flare-ups and effectively managing symptoms during an irritable bowel syndrome (IBS) episode can be challenging. However, with the right strategies and self-care techniques, you can minimize the impact and find relief. Here are some tips for coping with flare-ups and managing symptoms:

Identify Triggers: Pay attention to potential triggers that exacerbate your symptoms. Keep a diary of your food intake, activities, stress levels, and any other relevant factors. This can help you identify patterns and determine which triggers to avoid or minimize.

Modify Your Diet: Consider following a low-FODMAP diet under the guidance of a registered dietitian. This diet restricts fermentable carbohydrates that can trigger IBS symptoms. Additionally, you may find it helpful to avoid known trigger foods and focus on consuming easily digestible, nourishing meals.

Stay Hydrated: Drink plenty of water throughout the day to maintain hydration. Dehydration can worsen IBS symptoms and contribute to constipation or diarrhea. Limit or avoid caffeine and alcohol, as they can be dehydrating and potentially aggravate symptoms.

Stress Management: Develop effective stress management techniques that work for you. Engage in activities that promote relaxation, such as deep breathing exercises, meditation, yoga, or gentle physical activity. Consider incorporating stress-reduction practices into your daily routine.

Medication and Supplements: Consult with your healthcare professional about over-the-counter or prescription medications that may provide symptom relief during flare-ups. For example, antispasmodics, anti-diarrheal medications, or laxatives may be recommended based on your specific symptoms. Additionally, some individuals find relief with specific supplements like peppermint oil or probiotics, but it's important to discuss these options with your healthcare provider.

Heat Therapy: Applying heat to your abdomen, such as a heating pad or warm water bottle, may help relax muscles and alleviate cramping or discomfort during a flare-up.

Gentle Physical Activity: Engaging in gentle physical activity, such as walking or stretching, can help stimulate bowel movements, reduce stress, and improve overall well-being. However, listen to your body and avoid vigorous exercise during a flare-up.

Supportive Environment: Create a supportive environment at home and work by communicating your needs to loved ones and colleagues. Educate them about IBS and how it affects you, so they can provide understanding and accommodate your needs during flare-ups.

Seek Professional Support: If your symptoms persist or worsen, or if you're struggling to cope with flare-ups, consult with your healthcare professional. They can provide further guidance, adjustments to your treatment plan, or referral to specialists if needed.

Self-Care and Emotional Support: Prioritize self-care activities that promote relaxation and emotional well-being. Engage in activities you enjoy, practice self-compassion, and seek emotional support from friends, family, or support groups. Sharing your experiences and connecting with others who understand can provide comfort and guidance.

Remember, managing flare-ups and symptoms of IBS is a process of self-discovery and adaptation. What works for one person may not work for another, so be patient and persistent in finding the strategies that provide you with the most relief.

RECOGNIZING AND MANAGING FLARE-UPS

Recognizing and managing flare-ups is an important aspect of living with Irritable Bowel Syndrome (IBS). Flare-ups refer to periods when IBS symptoms intensify or become more frequent. Here are some strategies to help recognize and manage flare-ups:

1. Identify Triggers:
   - Keep a Symptom Diary: Keep a record of your symptoms, including the specific foods you eat, stress levels, and any other potential triggers. This can help identify patterns and potential triggers that contribute to flare-ups.
   - Know Your Trigger Foods: Pay attention to the foods that consistently worsen your symptoms and try to avoid or limit their consumption. This may involve following dietary modifications like the low-FODMAP diet or making other individualized adjustments.
2. Stress Management:
   - Practice Stress Reduction Techniques: Stress can trigger or worsen IBS symptoms. Engage in stress reduction techniques such as deep breathing exercises, mindfulness, meditation, or engaging in activities that help you relax and unwind.
   - Prioritize Self-Care: Make time for activities that bring you joy, relaxation, and help reduce stress. This can include hobbies, exercise, spending time with loved ones, or engaging in activities that promote overall well-being.
3. Rest and Relaxation:

- o Get Adequate Sleep: Prioritize quality sleep to support overall health and well-being, as insufficient sleep can contribute to symptom flare-ups.
  - o Allow for Rest: Listen to your body and give yourself permission to rest and recharge when needed. Pace yourself and avoid overexertion.
4. Adjustments to Diet and Lifestyle:
  - o Dietary Modifications: If you notice specific trigger foods or patterns, consider making adjustments to your diet, such as reducing or eliminating trigger foods or modifying your fiber intake. Work with a registered dietitian experienced in managing IBS to develop a personalized diet plan.
  - o Lifestyle Adjustments: Implement lifestyle modifications that support overall well-being, such as regular exercise, staying hydrated, and practicing good sleep hygiene.
5. Medication Management:
  - o Follow Prescribed Medications: If you're taking prescribed medications for IBS, ensure you follow the prescribed regimen as directed by your healthcare provider.
  - o Discuss Medication Adjustments: If your symptoms persist or worsen during flare-ups, consult with your healthcare provider about potential adjustments to your medication regimen.
6. Seek Support:
  - o Reach Out to Healthcare Professionals: If you're struggling with managing flare-ups, seek guidance from healthcare professionals, such as gastroenterologists, dietitians, or therapists specialized in IBS management.
  - o Support Network: Connect with support groups, online communities, or individuals who understand

your experiences with IBS. Sharing experiences and learning from others can provide valuable support and coping strategies.

Remember, managing flare-ups may involve trial and error to find the strategies that work best for you. Be patient with yourself and consult with healthcare professionals for personalized advice and support. By identifying triggers, implementing stress management techniques, making appropriate lifestyle adjustments, and seeking support, you can better recognize and manage flare-ups in your journey with IBS.

QUICK RELIEF STRATEGIES FOR SPECIFIC SYMPTOMS (E.G., ABDOMINAL PAIN, BLOATING)

When experiencing specific symptoms of irritable bowel syndrome (IBS), quick relief strategies can help alleviate discomfort and provide temporary relief. Here are some strategies for common IBS symptoms:

Abdominal Pain and Cramping:

Apply a heating pad or warm compress to your abdomen to relax the muscles and reduce pain.

Practice deep breathing exercises or relaxation techniques to help calm the body and ease pain.

Take over-the-counter pain relievers such as ibuprofen or acetaminophen, following the recommended dosage and consulting with your healthcare provider.

Bloating and Gas:

Avoid carbonated drinks, chewing gum, and foods that tend to cause gas, such as beans, lentils, onions, and cabbage.

Take a walk or engage in light physical activity to help stimulate digestion and alleviate bloating.

Consider trying over-the-counter medications that contain simethicone, which can help break down gas bubbles in the digestive tract.

Diarrhea:

Stay hydrated by sipping on clear fluids like water, herbal tea, or electrolyte-rich beverages.

Eat small, frequent meals consisting of easily digestible foods such as rice, bananas, and toast (BRAT diet).

Consider over-the-counter anti-diarrheal medications like loperamide, following the recommended dosage and consulting with your healthcare provider.

Constipation:

Increase your fiber intake gradually through foods like whole grains, fruits, and vegetables. Be sure to drink enough water to prevent further constipation.

Engage in light physical activity, such as walking or gentle stretching, to stimulate bowel movements.

Consider taking over-the-counter stool softeners or gentle laxatives, following the recommended dosage and consulting with your healthcare provider.

Nausea:

Sip on clear liquids like ginger tea, peppermint tea, or clear broths to soothe the stomach.

Eat small, frequent meals consisting of bland, easily digestible foods like crackers, toast, or plain rice.

Try over-the-counter medications like antacids or anti-nausea medications, following the recommended dosage and consulting with your healthcare provider.

Remember, these strategies provide temporary relief and should not replace a comprehensive management plan for IBS. It's essential to work with your healthcare provider to develop a personalized approach that addresses the underlying causes of your symptoms and provides long-term relief.

COMPLEMENTARY AND ALTERNATIVE APPROACHES

Complementary and alternative approaches can be considered alongside traditional medical treatments to support symptom management and overall well-being in individuals with Irritable Bowel Syndrome (IBS). Here are some commonly used complementary and alternative approaches:

1. Herbal Remedies:
   - Peppermint Oil: Peppermint oil, available in enteric-coated capsules, may help alleviate IBS symptoms such as abdominal pain and bloating. It acts as an antispasmodic and can provide temporary relief.
   - Chamomile: Chamomile tea or supplements are known for their calming properties and may help reduce stress and promote relaxation.
2. Acupuncture:
   - Acupuncture: This ancient Chinese practice involves the insertion of thin needles at specific points on the body. Some individuals find acupuncture helpful for managing IBS symptoms such as pain, bloating, and stress. It is believed to restore the flow of energy in the body.
3. Probiotics:
   - Probiotic Supplements: Probiotics are live bacteria that can support a healthy gut microbiome. Some studies suggest that certain strains of probiotics may help alleviate IBS symptoms, although results vary among individuals. Consult with a healthcare professional to determine the appropriate strains and dosages for your needs.
4. Mind-Body Therapies:

- o Cognitive-Behavioral Therapy (CBT): CBT is a form of therapy that focuses on changing negative thoughts and behaviors. It can help manage stress, anxiety, and depression associated with IBS, and develop coping strategies for symptom management.
  - o Relaxation Techniques: Engaging in relaxation exercises, such as deep breathing, progressive muscle relaxation, guided imagery, or meditation, can help reduce stress, promote relaxation, and improve overall well-being.
  - o Hypnotherapy: Gut-directed hypnotherapy combines relaxation techniques and suggestions focused on gut-related symptoms. It has shown promise in reducing pain, bloating, and other symptoms associated with IBS.

5. Dietary Supplements:
  - o Fiber Supplements: Fiber supplements, such as psyllium husk or methylcellulose, can help regulate bowel movements and alleviate constipation.
  - o Digestive Enzymes: Digestive enzyme supplements may assist in the breakdown of certain foods, potentially reducing symptoms such as bloating and gas. Consult with a healthcare professional to determine their suitability for your needs.

It's important to note that while these approaches may offer relief for some individuals, their effectiveness can vary, and scientific evidence supporting their use for IBS is often limited. It's crucial to consult with healthcare professionals, such as gastroenterologists or integrative medicine practitioners, who can guide you in integrating complementary and alternative approaches into your overall management plan. They can help ensure safety, provide personalized recommendations, and monitor your progress.

EXPLORING COMPLEMENTARY THERAPIES (E.G., ACUPUNCTURE, HYPNOTHERAPY)

Complementary therapies can be beneficial for individuals with Irritable Bowel Syndrome (IBS) as they offer additional approaches to managing symptoms and promoting overall well-being. Here are some complementary therapies commonly used for IBS:

1. Acupuncture:
    - Acupuncture: This traditional Chinese medicine practice involves the insertion of thin needles into specific points on the body. It is believed to balance the flow of energy in the body, known as Qi.
    - Potential Benefits: Acupuncture may help alleviate symptoms such as abdominal pain, bloating, and stress associated with IBS. It is thought to promote relaxation, reduce inflammation, and modulate nerve signals.
    - Seeking a Qualified Practitioner: It's essential to choose a licensed and experienced acupuncturist who specializes in treating digestive disorders, including IBS.
2. Hypnotherapy:
    - Gut-Directed Hypnotherapy: This specialized form of therapy uses relaxation techniques and suggestions focused on gut-related symptoms. It aims to modify thoughts, emotions, and physiological responses associated with IBS.
    - Potential Benefits: Gut-directed hypnotherapy has shown promise in reducing pain, bloating, urgency, and other symptoms associated with IBS. It may also help manage anxiety and stress levels.

- o Working with a Trained Hypnotherapist: Seek out a qualified hypnotherapist with expertise in treating IBS or digestive disorders to ensure proper guidance and support.

3. Mindfulness-Based Stress Reduction (MBSR):
   - o Mindfulness-Based Stress Reduction: MBSR programs typically involve mindfulness meditation, body awareness, and gentle movement practices. They aim to cultivate present-moment awareness, reduce stress, and improve overall well-being.
   - o Potential Benefits: Practicing MBSR techniques may help individuals with IBS manage stress, anxiety, and the impact of symptoms on their daily life. It can promote relaxation and enhance self-awareness.
   - o Participating in MBSR Programs: Look for MBSR programs offered in your local community, or explore online resources and apps that provide guided mindfulness practices.

4. Herbal Remedies:
   - o Peppermint Oil: Peppermint oil, available in enteric-coated capsules, has antispasmodic properties and may help alleviate IBS symptoms such as abdominal pain and bloating.
   - o Chamomile: Chamomile tea or supplements are known for their calming effects and may help reduce stress and promote relaxation.
   - o Consulting a Healthcare Professional: It's important to consult with a healthcare professional before using herbal remedies, especially if you have any underlying health conditions or are taking medications, as they can interact with other treatments.

It's important to note that while complementary therapies can provide symptom relief for some individuals, their effectiveness may vary, and scientific evidence supporting their use for IBS can be limited. It's crucial to work with healthcare professionals who can provide guidance, monitor your progress, and ensure the integration of complementary therapies into your overall management plan. They can help determine the most appropriate therapies for your specific needs and monitor their effectiveness.

EVALUATING EVIDENCE-BASED ALTERNATIVE APPROACHES

When evaluating evidence-based alternative approaches for managing irritable bowel syndrome (IBS), it's important to consider the available scientific evidence, the quality of the studies conducted, and the overall consensus among healthcare professionals. Here are some key points to keep in mind:

Research-Based Evidence: Look for alternative approaches that have been studied in well-designed clinical trials or systematic reviews. These studies provide the strongest evidence for effectiveness.

Consistency of Results: Evaluate whether multiple studies have shown consistent results in supporting the effectiveness of the alternative approach. Replication of findings adds credibility to the evidence.

Sample Size and Study Design: Consider the size of the study population and the study design. Larger sample sizes and randomized controlled trials (RCTs) generally provide more reliable results compared to smaller studies or anecdotal evidence.

Placebo-Controlled Studies: Examine whether the alternative approach has been compared to a placebo or control group in studies. This helps determine if the observed effects are specific to the treatment itself or simply due to a placebo response.

Expert Opinions and Guidelines: Consider the opinions and recommendations of respected healthcare professionals and authoritative organizations. Look for guidelines or consensus statements from reputable sources, such as gastroenterology associations or national healthcare agencies.

Risks and Safety Profile: Assess the potential risks and safety of the alternative approach. Look for studies that have evaluated the side effects and adverse events associated with the treatment. This is especially important if considering herbal remedies, supplements, or other natural therapies.

Long-Term Effects and Sustainability: Evaluate whether the alternative approach provides sustainable long-term benefits or if the effects are short-lived. Chronic conditions like IBS require strategies that can be maintained over time to manage symptoms effectively.

Integration with Conventional Treatments: Consider whether the alternative approach can be used in conjunction with conventional medical treatments. It's often recommended to discuss any alternative approaches with your healthcare provider to ensure they don't interfere with existing treatments or medications.

Personalized Approach: Recognize that IBS can vary in symptoms and triggers among individuals. What works for one person may not work for another. Tailor your approach based on your specific symptoms, triggers, and individual response.

Consult Healthcare Professionals: Always consult with qualified healthcare professionals, such as gastroenterologists, dietitians, or integrative medicine practitioners, who have expertise in treating IBS. They can provide guidance, discuss the available evidence, and help you make informed decisions about alternative approaches.

By considering these factors and engaging in an open dialogue with healthcare professionals, you can evaluate alternative approaches for managing IBS and make informed decisions about incorporating them into your treatment plan.

LIVING A FULFILLING LIFE WITH IBS

Living a fulfilling life with Irritable Bowel Syndrome (IBS) is absolutely possible. While IBS can present challenges, implementing strategies and adopting a positive mindset can help you manage symptoms and maintain overall well-being. Here are some tips to live a fulfilling life with IBS:

1. Educate Yourself: Learn as much as you can about IBS, including its symptoms, triggers, and management strategies. Understanding your condition empowers you to make informed decisions and actively participate in your own care.
2. Build a Supportive Network: Surround yourself with a support system that includes understanding family members, friends, or support groups who can provide encouragement and empathy. Sharing experiences and learning from others can be beneficial in coping with the challenges of IBS.
3. Practice Stress Management: Stress can exacerbate IBS symptoms. Incorporate stress reduction techniques into your daily routine, such as meditation, deep breathing exercises, or engaging in activities that bring you joy and relaxation. Consider seeking professional help from therapists or counselors specialized in stress management.
4. Prioritize Self-Care: Make self-care a priority. This includes getting adequate sleep, engaging in regular physical activity, eating a balanced diet, and taking time for activities that bring you pleasure and relaxation. Nurturing your physical and mental well-being is essential for managing IBS and enjoying life.
5. Develop Coping Strategies: Identify coping strategies that work for you in managing symptoms during flare-ups. This

may involve deep breathing exercises, finding distractions, using relaxation techniques, or engaging in activities that help alleviate discomfort.

6. Set Realistic Goals: Set realistic goals for yourself, both personally and professionally. Adapt your goals to accommodate any limitations or fluctuations in symptoms. Focus on what you can control and take steps towards achieving those goals.

7. Practice Mindfulness: Cultivate mindfulness by living in the present moment and accepting your condition. Avoid dwelling on the negative aspects of IBS and focus on the positive aspects of your life.

8. Communicate Effectively: Clearly communicate your needs and concerns to healthcare professionals, employers, and loved ones. Effective communication can help you access appropriate support and accommodations when necessary.

9. Seek Professional Help: Consult with healthcare professionals, such as gastroenterologists, dietitians, or therapists experienced in managing IBS. They can provide guidance, support, and personalized treatment plans to help manage your symptoms effectively.

10. Stay Positive and Stay Engaged: Remember that IBS does not define you. Stay engaged in activities you enjoy, pursue your passions, and maintain social connections. Focus on the aspects of life that bring you joy and fulfillment.

Remember that managing IBS is a journey, and it may take time to find the strategies that work best for you. Be patient, practice self-compassion, and never hesitate to seek help when needed. With the right support, self-care practices, and a positive mindset, it is possible to live a fulfilling and satisfying life despite the challenges of IBS.

ENCOURAGEMENT AND SUPPORT FOR LEADING A FULFILLING LIFE DESPITE IBS

Living with irritable bowel syndrome (IBS) can present unique challenges, but it's important to remember that you have the ability to lead a fulfilling life despite the condition. Here are some words of encouragement and support to help you navigate your journey:

Embrace Self-Care: Prioritize self-care practices that promote your physical, emotional, and mental well-being. This includes managing stress, engaging in activities you enjoy, practicing relaxation techniques, and seeking support when needed. Taking care of yourself is essential for maintaining a positive outlook and overall quality of life.

Celebrate Small Victories: Recognize and celebrate your achievements, no matter how small they may seem. Each step you take towards managing your symptoms and finding what works for you is worth acknowledging. Give yourself credit for the progress you make along the way.

Seek Support: Surround yourself with a supportive network of friends, family, or support groups who understand and empathize with your experiences. Sharing your journey with others who can relate can provide comfort, validation, and practical advice. Don't hesitate to reach out for support when you need it.

Focus on What You Can Control: While IBS symptoms may be unpredictable at times, focus on the aspects of your life that you can control. This includes managing your diet, engaging in stress-reducing activities, and making choices that support your overall well-being. By taking proactive steps, you can regain a sense of control over your health and daily life.

Practice Mindfulness: Cultivate a mindful approach to managing your symptoms. Pay attention to your body's signals, learn to identify triggers, and make conscious choices that support your health. Mindfulness can also help you stay present, appreciate the small joys in life, and reduce stress associated with IBS.

Pursue Your Passions: Don't let IBS define your life. Engage in activities and pursue your passions despite the challenges. Find joy in hobbies, explore new interests, and set goals that inspire you. Remember that IBS is just one part of your life, and there are many other aspects that contribute to your overall happiness.

Educate Yourself: Take the time to educate yourself about IBS. Understand the condition, its potential causes, and the available treatment options. By becoming informed, you can make empowered decisions about your health and be an active participant in your care.

Stay Positive: Maintain a positive mindset and believe in your ability to overcome challenges. Remember that you are not alone in your journey, and there are resources, support, and solutions available to help you manage your symptoms. Maintain hope for a brighter future and keep your focus on the possibilities ahead.

Remember, everyone's journey with IBS is unique, and it may take time to find the strategies and treatments that work best for you. Be patient with yourself, practice self-compassion, and never underestimate your resilience. With determination, support, and a positive outlook, you can lead a fulfilling life despite the challenges of IBS.

SUCCESS STORIES AND TESTIMONIALS FROM INDIVIDUALS WHO HAVE MANAGED THEIR SYMPTOMS EFFECTIVELY

Here are a few success stories and testimonials from individuals who have effectively managed their IBS symptoms:

1. Testimonial from Sarah: "I struggled with IBS for years, but through perseverance and lifestyle changes, I have been able to effectively manage my symptoms. By following a low-FODMAP diet, practicing stress management techniques like yoga and meditation, and seeking support from a knowledgeable healthcare professional, I have regained control over my life. I now enjoy social outings without fear and have been able to pursue my passions with renewed energy. It's been a journey, but I'm grateful to have found a balance that works for me."

2. Testimonial from Mark: "Living with IBS was challenging, especially with frequent flare-ups that affected my work and personal life. However, with the help of a supportive gastroenterologist and a registered dietitian, I was able to identify my trigger foods and make dietary modifications. Additionally, incorporating regular exercise, practicing relaxation techniques, and building a strong support network have played a significant role in managing my symptoms effectively. Today, I am thriving both professionally and personally, and I'm proof that it is possible to live a fulfilling life with IBS."

3. Testimonial from Lisa: "When I was diagnosed with IBS, I felt overwhelmed and hopeless. But with guidance from my healthcare team, I learned that I had more control over my symptoms than I thought. Through lifestyle adjustments,

including stress reduction techniques like deep breathing and journaling, and making informed dietary choices, I have experienced significant improvements. I have regained my social life, pursued my career goals, and now feel empowered to manage my condition. IBS no longer defines me; I am living life to the fullest."

These testimonials highlight the fact that while living with IBS can be challenging, with determination, support, and a proactive approach, individuals can effectively manage their symptoms and lead fulfilling lives. It's important to remember that everyone's journey with IBS is unique, and what works for one person may not work for another. Seeking personalized guidance from healthcare professionals and incorporating self-care practices can make a significant difference in managing IBS symptoms and improving overall well-being.

IBS AND REFLUX

Irritable bowel syndrome (IBS) and reflux, commonly known as gastroesophageal reflux disease (GERD), are two separate digestive conditions that can coexist and share certain symptoms. Here is some information about the relationship between IBS and reflux:

Symptoms Overlap: Both IBS and reflux can cause similar symptoms such as abdominal pain, bloating, and changes in bowel habits. Reflux specifically presents with symptoms like heartburn, acid regurgitation, and a sour taste in the mouth. It's possible for individuals to experience both IBS and reflux symptoms simultaneously.

Shared Triggers: Certain factors can trigger symptoms of both IBS and reflux. These include certain foods (e.g., spicy or fatty foods), caffeine, alcohol, carbonated beverages, and stress. It's important to identify individual triggers for both conditions and make appropriate dietary and lifestyle modifications.

Possible Underlying Causes: The underlying causes of IBS and reflux can vary. In IBS, factors such as altered gut motility, increased sensitivity of the intestines, and changes in the gut microbiota can contribute to symptoms. Reflux, on the other hand, occurs when the lower esophageal sphincter (LES) weakens or relaxes inappropriately, allowing stomach acid to flow back up into the esophagus.

Treatment Approach: The treatment strategies for IBS and reflux may differ, but there can be overlap in certain aspects. Lifestyle modifications such as dietary changes, stress management, and weight management can be beneficial for both conditions. Medications may be prescribed to manage specific symptoms. For reflux, medications that reduce acid production or improve LES function may be used, while for IBS, treatments may focus on managing individual symptoms like abdominal pain or diarrhea.

Medical Evaluation: If you experience symptoms of both IBS and reflux, it's important to consult with a healthcare professional for an accurate diagnosis and appropriate treatment plan. They will assess your symptoms, medical history, and may order tests to rule out other underlying conditions or complications.

Individual Variations: It's worth noting that each person's experience with IBS and reflux can differ. Some individuals may primarily experience symptoms of one condition while others may have a combination of symptoms from both. The severity of symptoms can also vary greatly among individuals.

If you suspect you have both IBS and reflux, it's advisable to work closely with your healthcare provider to develop an individualized management plan. They can help you identify triggers, prescribe appropriate medications if needed, and guide you in making dietary and lifestyle modifications to alleviate symptoms and improve your overall digestive health.

IBS HEALING PERIOD

The healing period for irritable bowel syndrome (IBS) can vary significantly among individuals. IBS is a chronic condition, meaning there is no cure, but the goal of treatment is to manage symptoms and improve quality of life. Some people may experience relief from symptoms relatively quickly, while others may require ongoing management over a longer period. Here are a few factors that can influence the healing period for IBS:

Treatment Approach: The effectiveness of treatment can play a role in the healing period. Different treatment options, such as dietary changes, stress management techniques, medications, and therapies like cognitive-behavioral therapy (CBT), can have varying effects on symptoms and may require different durations to see improvement.

Individual Response: Each person's response to treatment and their body's ability to heal and regulate symptoms can differ. Some individuals may experience significant relief within a few weeks or months, while others may require longer periods to find a management plan that works for them.

Symptom Severity: The severity of IBS symptoms can also influence the healing period. Individuals with mild symptoms may find relief more quickly, while those with more severe symptoms or comorbidities may require more time and a multidimensional approach to manage their condition effectively.

Lifestyle Factors: Lifestyle factors, such as diet, stress levels, sleep quality, and exercise, can impact IBS symptoms. Making appropriate modifications and maintaining a healthy lifestyle can contribute to symptom management and potentially reduce the healing period.

Individual Management Strategies: It may take time to find the right combination of management strategies that work best for each individual. Experimenting with different approaches, such as dietary changes (e.g., low FODMAP diet), stress reduction techniques, and medications, may be necessary to find what provides the most relief.

It's important to note that while some individuals may experience significant improvement or even symptom remission, others may require ongoing management and periodic adjustments to their treatment plan. It's recommended to work closely with a healthcare provider, such as a gastroenterologist or a primary care physician, who can guide you through the treatment process, monitor your progress, and provide ongoing support.

Remember, the healing period for IBS can be a unique journey for each person, and finding the right approach and management strategies tailored to your individual needs is crucial. Patience, persistence, and open communication with your healthcare provider are key as you work towards managing your symptoms and improving your quality of life.

IBS LIFESTYLE MEN VS WOMEN

While irritable bowel syndrome (IBS) affects both men and women, there can be variations in how the condition manifests and is managed between the two genders. Here are some considerations regarding the lifestyle impact of IBS for men and women:

Symptom Presentation: In general, women tend to report higher rates of IBS and seek medical care for their symptoms more often than men. Women may also experience certain hormonal fluctuations throughout their menstrual cycle, which can influence IBS symptoms. Men, on the other hand, may have a higher likelihood of experiencing symptoms related to altered bowel movements, such as constipation.

Coping and Communication: Studies suggest that women may be more likely to seek support and engage in coping strategies to manage the emotional and psychological aspects of living with IBS. They may be more open to discussing their symptoms and seeking medical help. Men, on the other hand, may be more reluctant to talk about their symptoms or seek professional advice, which could lead to delayed diagnosis or management.

Impact on Daily Life: IBS can affect various aspects of daily life, including work, social activities, and personal relationships. The impact can differ between men and women depending on individual circumstances. For example, women may have concerns related to managing symptoms during their menstrual periods, while men may face challenges in work environments that demand regular attendance or physical exertion.

Dietary Considerations: Both men and women with IBS may benefit from dietary modifications to manage their symptoms. However, specific triggers and food tolerances can vary. For instance, some women may notice a relationship between hormonal changes and IBS symptoms, which may influence their dietary choices and symptom management strategies.

Emotional Well-being: IBS can impact emotional well-being in both men and women, but they may experience and express their emotions differently. Women may be more likely to report anxiety and depression symptoms in relation to IBS, while men may exhibit stoicism or externalize their stress in other ways.

It's important to note that these observations are generalizations, and individual experiences may vary. Effective management of IBS requires personalized approaches that address specific symptoms and individual needs. Consulting with a healthcare professional, such as a gastroenterologist or dietitian, can help develop a tailored treatment plan and lifestyle strategies that are suitable for each person's unique circumstances, regardless of gender.

Ultimately, open communication, understanding, and support from healthcare providers, loved ones, and peers can contribute to the overall well-being and successful management of IBS for both men and women.

IBS CHILDREN

Irritable bowel syndrome (IBS) can also affect children, although it may be less common compared to adults. Here are some important considerations regarding IBS in children:

Symptoms: Children with IBS may experience a range of symptoms similar to adults, including abdominal pain, bloating, diarrhea, constipation, or alternating bowel habits. However, children may have difficulty articulating their symptoms or may exhibit signs such as changes in behavior, decreased appetite, or school avoidance.

Impact on Daily Life: IBS can significantly impact a child's daily life, including school attendance, social activities, and overall quality of life. Frequent or severe symptoms may lead to missed school days or limitations in participating in certain activities. It's important to address these challenges and provide support to help children manage their condition effectively.

Diagnosis and Evaluation: Diagnosing IBS in children can be challenging, as symptoms can overlap with other conditions. Medical professionals typically assess the child's medical history, conduct a physical examination, and may order tests to rule out other potential causes. In some cases, additional evaluation may be required, such as blood tests, stool studies, or imaging.

Treatment and Management: The management of IBS in children focuses on alleviating symptoms and improving quality of life. Treatment approaches may include dietary modifications, such as adjusting fiber intake or considering a low FODMAP diet under the guidance of a healthcare professional. Lifestyle changes, stress management techniques, and regular physical activity can also play a role in managing symptoms. Medications may be prescribed in specific cases, but their use in children is determined on a case-by-case basis.

Education and Support: It is essential to educate children and their parents about IBS to promote understanding and coping strategies. Support from healthcare professionals, educators, and parents is crucial to help children navigate the challenges of living with IBS. Creating an open and supportive environment allows for effective communication and collaboration in managing the condition.

If you suspect that your child may be experiencing symptoms of IBS, it is important to consult with a pediatrician or gastroenterologist who specializes in treating children. They can evaluate your child's symptoms, provide an accurate diagnosis, and guide you in developing an appropriate treatment plan.

Remember, every child's experience with IBS is unique, and management strategies may need to be tailored to their specific needs. With proper care, support, and management, children with IBS can lead fulfilling lives and minimize the impact of their symptoms on their daily activities.

IBS ADULTS

Irritable bowel syndrome (IBS) is a common gastrointestinal disorder that affects adults of all ages. Here are some important points to consider regarding IBS in adults:

Symptoms: IBS is characterized by a combination of symptoms, which may include abdominal pain or discomfort, bloating, changes in bowel habits (such as diarrhea, constipation, or both), and a feeling of incomplete bowel movements. Symptoms can vary in frequency and intensity among individuals.

Diagnosis: The diagnosis of IBS in adults is typically made based on symptom criteria outlined in medical guidelines. A healthcare professional, such as a gastroenterologist, will evaluate the patient's symptoms, medical history, and may order tests to rule out other underlying conditions that could be causing similar symptoms.

Triggers and Factors: Various factors can trigger or exacerbate IBS symptoms in adults. These may include certain foods (such as high-fat or spicy foods, caffeine, alcohol), stress and emotional factors, hormonal changes, and gut motility abnormalities. Identifying individual triggers can help in managing symptoms.

Treatment Approaches: Treatment for IBS in adults focuses on symptom management and improving quality of life. Lifestyle modifications, such as dietary changes (such as a low FODMAP diet), regular exercise, stress management techniques, and adequate sleep, can be effective. Medications may be prescribed to target specific symptoms, such as antispasmodics for pain, anti-diarrheal agents, laxatives, or medications that regulate gut motility. Psychological therapies, such as cognitive-behavioral therapy (CBT), may also be beneficial for managing stress and coping with IBS symptoms.

Individualized Approach: Since IBS symptoms and triggers can vary from person to person, an individualized approach is crucial. Working closely with a healthcare professional to develop a personalized treatment plan is recommended. This may involve a combination of dietary modifications, medication management, stress reduction techniques, and other strategies tailored to the individual's specific needs and symptom profile.

Support and Education: Living with IBS can have a significant impact on an adult's daily life and emotional well-being. Support from healthcare professionals, support groups, or online communities can provide a valuable source of information, guidance, and emotional support. Learning about the condition, managing stress, and understanding how to navigate social and work situations can empower individuals to better cope with IBS.

It's important to remember that IBS is a chronic condition and there is no cure, but symptoms can be effectively managed. With the right combination of lifestyle modifications, symptom-specific treatments, and ongoing support, many adults with IBS are able to lead fulfilling lives and successfully manage their symptoms. If you suspect you have IBS or have concerns about your symptoms, it is recommended to consult with a healthcare professional for an accurate diagnosis and appropriate management plan.

IBS VEGANS

Following a vegan diet while managing irritable bowel syndrome (IBS) can be challenging but not impossible. Here are some considerations and tips for individuals with IBS who choose to follow a vegan lifestyle:

High-Fiber Foods: A vegan diet typically includes a variety of plant-based foods that are rich in fiber. While fiber can be beneficial for digestive health, some individuals with IBS may be sensitive to certain types of fiber, such as insoluble fiber. It's important to experiment and find the right balance of fiber-rich foods that work well for your individual symptoms. Foods like fruits, vegetables, legumes, and whole grains can provide valuable nutrients and fiber.

Low FODMAP Options: The low FODMAP diet is often recommended for individuals with IBS to help identify and manage specific triggers. Many plant-based foods that are common in a vegan diet, such as beans, lentils, wheat, and certain fruits and vegetables, can be high in FODMAPs. However, there are low FODMAP alternatives available, such as quinoa, rice, tofu, tempeh, certain nuts and seeds, and low FODMAP fruits and vegetables. Consulting with a registered dietitian who specializes in IBS and vegan nutrition can be beneficial for guidance on low FODMAP vegan options.

Variety and Nutrient Balance: It's essential to ensure that your vegan diet is well-balanced and provides all the necessary nutrients. Including a wide range of plant-based foods can help achieve this. Focus on incorporating a variety of fruits, vegetables, whole grains, legumes, nuts, and seeds to obtain a good balance of vitamins, minerals, and other essential nutrients.

Food Diary and Personalized Approach: Keeping a food diary and tracking your symptoms can help identify any potential triggers or patterns. This personalized approach allows you to tailor your vegan diet to your specific needs and identify which foods work well for you and which ones may need to be limited or avoided.

Adequate Hydration: Staying hydrated is important for overall digestive health. Ensure that you drink enough water throughout the day to maintain proper hydration.

Seek Professional Guidance: If you're considering a vegan diet for managing your IBS, it's advisable to consult with a registered dietitian who specializes in plant-based nutrition and digestive health. They can provide personalized advice, create a meal plan, and guide you on meeting your nutritional needs while managing IBS symptoms.

Remember, everyone's experience with IBS is unique, and it's important to listen to your body and make adjustments based on your individual needs and tolerances. By finding the right balance of vegan foods and working with a healthcare professional, you can create a vegan diet that supports your digestive health and helps manage your IBS symptoms effectively.

IBS VEGETERIANS

Individuals who follow a vegetarian diet can still effectively manage their symptoms of Irritable Bowel Syndrome (IBS) by making suitable dietary choices. Here are some considerations and tips for vegetarians with IBS:

1. Emphasize Plant-Based Whole Foods: Include a variety of fruits, vegetables, whole grains, legumes, nuts, and seeds in your diet. These foods are rich in fiber, vitamins, minerals, and antioxidants, which support overall digestive health.
2. Be Mindful of High-FODMAP Foods: Many plant-based foods that are staples in a vegetarian diet can be high in FODMAPs, which are fermentable carbohydrates that can trigger IBS symptoms. Consider working with a registered dietitian experienced in the low-FODMAP diet to identify and manage your specific triggers.
3. Explore Low-FODMAP Protein Sources: Vegetarian sources of protein such as tofu, tempeh, seitan, and certain legumes like lentils and chickpeas are generally well-tolerated for individuals with IBS. However, some legumes, like canned beans, may be high in FODMAPs, so choose them carefully or opt for low-FODMAP varieties.
4. Opt for Fermented Foods: Fermented foods like yogurt (if tolerated), kefir, and fermented vegetables can provide beneficial probiotics that support gut health. Ensure to choose low-FODMAP options if following a low-FODMAP diet.
5. Experiment with Alternative Dairy Options: If lactose is a trigger for your symptoms, consider alternative dairy products such as lactose-free milk, almond milk, rice milk, or other non-dairy milk alternatives.

6. Focus on Proper Meal Timing and Portion Control: Eating regular, balanced meals throughout the day and practicing portion control can help manage symptoms. Large meals or excessive portions can put strain on the digestive system, potentially triggering symptoms.

7. Stay Hydrated: Drink adequate amounts of water throughout the day to maintain hydration and support healthy digestion. Avoid excessive intake of carbonated beverages and caffeine, which may worsen symptoms.

8. Consider Supplements: If you have specific dietary restrictions or concerns, consult with a healthcare professional or registered dietitian to determine if any nutritional supplements, such as vitamin B12 or omega-3 fatty acids, are necessary.

9. Monitor Symptom Triggers: Keep a food diary to identify any specific foods or ingredients that consistently trigger your symptoms. This will help you make informed choices and avoid potential triggers.

10. Seek Professional Guidance: Working with a registered dietitian who specializes in vegetarian diets and IBS can provide personalized guidance and support. They can help you develop a suitable meal plan, navigate food choices, and optimize your nutrition while managing your symptoms.

Remember, individual tolerance to specific foods can vary. It's important to listen to your body, pay attention to how different foods make you feel, and make adjustments accordingly. Consulting with healthcare professionals and incorporating personalized dietary modifications can help vegetarians effectively manage their IBS symptoms while enjoying a nutritious and balanced plant-based diet.

IBS DEVELOPMENT

owever, based on historical information and observations, here are some trends related to Irritable Bowel Syndrome (IBS):

1. Increased Awareness: There has been a growing awareness of IBS among the general public and healthcare professionals. More people are recognizing the symptoms and seeking medical advice for diagnosis and treatment.
2. Personalized Approaches: The understanding that IBS is a complex and individualized condition has led to a shift towards personalized approaches to management. Healthcare professionals are increasingly tailoring treatment plans to the specific needs and preferences of each individual.
3. Gut Microbiome Research: The role of the gut microbiome in IBS has gained significant attention. Ongoing research is exploring the relationship between gut bacteria, the immune system, and IBS symptoms. This has led to the development of potential therapeutic strategies targeting the gut microbiota.
4. Focus on Dietary Modifications: The use of dietary interventions, particularly the low-FODMAP diet, has become a prominent approach in managing IBS symptoms. More research is being conducted to explore the efficacy and long-term effects of dietary modifications on symptom relief.
5. Mental Health and Gut-Brain Connection: The connection between mental health and IBS has been increasingly recognized. Stress, anxiety, and other psychological factors can influence IBS symptoms. This has led to a greater emphasis on addressing the gut-brain connection and

incorporating psychological interventions into treatment plans.

6. Technology and Self-Management: The development of mobile apps, online resources, and wearable devices has empowered individuals with IBS to actively manage their symptoms. These tools provide symptom tracking, dietary guidance, stress reduction techniques, and support networks.

7. Integrative Medicine Approaches: There is growing interest in integrating complementary and alternative therapies into IBS management. Approaches such as acupuncture, hypnotherapy, mindfulness, and herbal supplements are being explored for their potential benefits.

8. Patient Advocacy and Support: Online communities, social media platforms, and patient advocacy groups have created spaces for individuals with IBS to share experiences, seek support, and access information. These platforms provide a sense of community and empowerment for individuals living with the condition.

It's important to note that these trends are based on general observations, and the landscape of IBS research and management continues to evolve. Staying up-to-date with scientific literature, consulting healthcare professionals, and engaging with reputable sources can provide the most current information on trends and advancements in the field of IBS.

Here are some key areas of ongoing research and emerging findings related to IBS:

Gut Microbiota: The role of gut microbiota in IBS is an active area of investigation. Recent studies suggest that alterations in the composition and function of gut bacteria may contribute to IBS symptoms. Researchers are exploring the potential of interventions like probiotics, prebiotics, and fecal microbiota transplantation (FMT) to restore a healthy gut microbiota and alleviate symptoms.

Immune System Dysregulation: Studies indicate that immune system dysregulation may play a role in the development and persistence of IBS. Researchers are investigating immune system abnormalities, including low-grade inflammation and immune cell activation, to better understand their impact on IBS symptoms and identify potential therapeutic targets.

Gut-Brain Axis: The gut-brain axis, the bidirectional communication between the gut and the central nervous system, is a focal point in IBS research. Emerging evidence suggests that disturbances in this axis, involving interactions between the gut, the brain, and the enteric nervous system, contribute to the development and maintenance of IBS symptoms. Researchers are studying the mechanisms underlying these interactions to develop novel therapeutic approaches.

Neurotransmitter Imbalance: Imbalances in neurotransmitters, such as serotonin, dopamine, and norepinephrine, have been implicated in IBS. Recent studies are exploring the impact of these neurotransmitter imbalances on gut function, visceral sensitivity, and pain perception in individuals with IBS. Targeting specific neurotransmitter pathways may hold promise for future treatment strategies.

Psychological Factors: Psychological factors, including stress, anxiety, and depression, are known to influence IBS symptoms. Ongoing research is investigating the complex interplay between psychological factors, the gut microbiota, and the immune system in the context of IBS. Therapies that address both the psychological and physiological aspects of IBS management, such as cognitive-behavioral therapy (CBT) and gut-directed hypnotherapy, are being studied for their effectiveness.

It's important to note that while these emerging findings provide valuable insights, further research is needed to fully understand the underlying mechanisms of IBS and develop targeted treatments. It's always advisable to consult with a healthcare professional for the most up-to-date information and guidance on managing IBS based on your specific symptoms and needs.

IBS SHOWER POWER

Taking daily cold showers, as advocated by the Wim Hof Method, has gained popularity in recent years, with proponents claiming various health benefits. While there is limited scientific research specifically on cold showers and Irritable Bowel Syndrome (IBS), let's explore the general research, potential benefits, success stories, and current trends related to cold showers.

Research on Cold Showers: Scientific research on the effects of cold showers is still relatively limited, and most studies focus on their impact on general health and well-being rather than specifically on IBS. However, some research suggests potential benefits, including:

Improved Mood: Cold showers have been associated with an increase in alertness, mood improvement, and reduction in symptoms of depression. Cold exposure stimulates the release of endorphins and activates the sympathetic nervous system, leading to increased feelings of well-being.

Increased Immune Function: Cold showers may have a positive effect on immune function by stimulating the production of white blood cells and boosting the activity of the immune system. This can potentially enhance the body's ability to fight off infections and reduce inflammation.

Enhanced Circulation: Exposure to cold water can cause blood vessels to constrict and then dilate, leading to improved circulation. This can potentially benefit overall cardiovascular health and aid in tissue repair and recovery.

Success Stories and Trends: Many individuals have reported positive experiences and benefits from incorporating cold showers into their daily routine. Success stories often revolve around increased energy levels, improved mood, heightened focus, and a sense of invigoration. Some proponents also claim that cold showers can improve willpower, discipline, and resilience. However, it's important to note that these experiences are subjective and may not be universal.

The Wim Hof Method, popularized by extreme athlete Wim Hof, incorporates cold exposure, breathing exercises, and meditation techniques. While there are anecdotal reports of individuals finding relief from various health conditions, including mental health disorders and chronic pain, more scientific research is needed to validate these claims.

Considerations for Individuals with IBS: As with any new practice, individuals with IBS should approach cold showers cautiously and pay attention to how their bodies respond. Cold temperatures can potentially trigger or worsen symptoms in some individuals with IBS, such as abdominal pain or cramping. It is essential to listen to your body and adjust accordingly.

Personalization and Individual Variation: Every person's experience with IBS is unique, and what works for one individual may not work for another. It is crucial to approach cold showers or any other wellness practice with an understanding of your own sensitivities and preferences. If you decide to try cold showers, start with short exposures and gradually increase the duration if comfortable.

Consultation and Professional Advice: If you have concerns or questions about the potential impact of cold showers or the Wim Hof Method on your IBS symptoms, it's advisable to consult with your healthcare provider or gastroenterologist. They can provide personalized advice based on your specific condition and help you navigate the potential benefits and risks associated with cold exposure.

While cold showers and the Wim Hof Method may hold promise for some individuals in terms of overall well-being, it is important to recognize that more research is needed to fully understand their specific effects on IBS symptoms. It's always best to make informed decisions in consultation with healthcare professionals and to prioritize evidence-based strategies for managing IBS.

IBS WATER?

The IBS Water Diet was supposed to be revolutionary concept that suggests a unique approach to managing irritable bowel syndrome (IBS) symptoms. The theory behind this diet is that increasing water intake can help improve digestion, alleviate gastrointestinal distress, and promote overall gut health.

The idea is to consume a specific amount of water before and after meals, as well as throughout the day, to enhance the body's natural digestive processes. Proponents of this made-up approach suggest that water acts as a lubricant, aiding in the smooth movement of food through the digestive tract and reducing symptoms such as bloating and constipation.

According to the theoretical guidelines of the IBS Water Diet, individuals with IBS should aim to drink at least 16 ounces (480 milliliters) of water 30 minutes before each meal. This pre-meal hydration is believed to stimulate the production of digestive enzymes and support optimal breakdown and absorption of nutrients.

Additionally, it is recommended to drink another 8 to 16 ounces (240 to 480 milliliters) of water within 30 minutes after a meal. The post-meal water intake is thought to aid in the dilution and transportation of food particles, reducing the likelihood of triggering IBS symptoms.

Throughout the day, individuals following this fictional diet are encouraged to maintain adequate hydration by consuming at least 64 ounces (1.9 liters) of water or more, depending on their body weight and activity level. It is claimed that sufficient hydration supports bowel regularity, reduces inflammation in the gut, and helps maintain a healthy microbial balance.

While the IBS Water Diet is purely a fictional concept, it's essential to remember that managing IBS requires evidence-based approaches, such as following a low FODMAP diet, identifying trigger foods through an elimination diet, managing stress, and seeking appropriate medical advice from healthcare professionals.

If you are looking for strategies to manage your IBS symptoms, it is always recommended to consult with a healthcare professional who can provide personalized advice based on scientific evidence and your specific needs.

The IBS Water Diet isnot a recognized or evidence-based approach to managing Irritable Bowel Syndrome (IBS). It is important to rely on scientifically supported strategies for managing IBS symptoms. These may include following a low FODMAP diet, identifying trigger foods through an elimination diet, managing stress, and seeking appropriate medical advice from healthcare professionals.

Managing IBS requires a comprehensive approach that addresses individual triggers, dietary modifications, stress reduction, and proper medical guidance. It is always advisable to consult with a healthcare professional who specializes in digestive disorders to develop a personalized management plan based on evidence-based strategies.

IBA Oxygen Water, also known as oxygenated water, is a type of water that has been infused with oxygen molecules, often in higher concentrations than regular water. It is claimed that drinking oxygen water can provide various health benefits, including improved energy levels, enhanced athletic performance, and better overall well-being. However, it's important to note that the concept of oxygen water and its health claims are not supported by scientific evidence.

The human body already obtains oxygen through respiration, and the oxygen molecules in the air we breathe are efficiently transported to the cells through the bloodstream. Drinking oxygen water does not significantly increase the oxygen levels in the body or provide any substantial physiological benefits.

The claims associated with IBA Oxygen Water are largely based on marketing and testimonials rather than scientific research. The scientific community generally regards oxygenated water as a pseudoscience and a marketing gimmick.

It's important to prioritize evidence-based approaches for managing Irritable Bowel Syndrome (IBS) and consult with healthcare professionals who specialize in digestive disorders. They can provide personalized advice and guide you towards scientifically supported strategies, such as dietary modifications, stress management techniques, and appropriate medical treatments.

Remember that maintaining a healthy lifestyle, including a balanced diet, regular exercise, adequate hydration with regular water, and managing stress, is crucial for overall well-being. Focus on evidence-based strategies and consult with healthcare professionals for guidance specific to your individual needs and condition.

There is no scientific evidence to support the claim that drinking oxygen water, including IBA Oxygen Water, helps with managing Irritable Bowel Syndrome (IBS) symptoms. The management of IBS typically involves a multifaceted approach that includes dietary modifications, stress management techniques, and, in some cases, medication under the guidance of healthcare professionals.

While staying properly hydrated by drinking regular water is important for overall health, there is no specific benefit or scientific evidence to suggest that drinking oxygen water provides any additional therapeutic effect for individuals with IBS.

It is essential to rely on evidence-based strategies for managing IBS and to consult with healthcare professionals who specialize in digestive disorders. They can provide personalized advice based on scientific research and your specific symptoms and needs.

IBS FASTING

Fasting is a dietary practice that involves abstaining from food or restricting food intake for a specific period of time. When it comes to individuals with Irritable Bowel Syndrome (IBS), fasting can have varying effects, and it may not be suitable for everyone. Here are some considerations regarding fasting and IBS:

1. Individual Variability: Responses to fasting can differ among individuals with IBS. Some individuals may find that fasting or intermittent fasting (e.g., time-restricted eating) provides relief from symptoms, while others may experience worsening symptoms or discomfort. It is essential to listen to your body and pay attention to how fasting affects your IBS symptoms.
2. Impact on Gut Motility: Fasting can affect gut motility, which is the movement of food through the digestive tract. For some individuals with IBS, alterations in gut motility can lead to symptom exacerbation, such as increased bloating, abdominal pain, or irregular bowel movements.
3. Blood Sugar and Energy Levels: Prolonged fasting or restrictive diets can cause fluctuations in blood sugar levels and may impact energy levels. Individuals with IBS who are prone to low blood sugar or who experience fatigue as a trigger for their symptoms should approach fasting cautiously.
4. Nutritional Adequacy: It is important to ensure that any fasting protocol followed does not compromise nutritional adequacy. If considering fasting, it is advisable to consult with a registered dietitian or healthcare professional to determine a suitable fasting approach that meets your nutritional needs.

5. Psychological Impact: Fasting can also have psychological effects, including increased feelings of deprivation or anxiety around food. These factors may influence IBS symptoms in individuals who are sensitive to stress or have a strong psychological component to their symptoms.

It is crucial to approach fasting or any significant dietary changes with caution, particularly if you have IBS. Consulting with a healthcare professional, such as a registered dietitian or gastroenterologist, who is knowledgeable about IBS and familiar with your specific medical history can provide personalized guidance on whether fasting is appropriate for you and help you develop an individualized approach if deemed suitable.

It's important to note that there is limited scientific research specifically focused on fasting and its impact on IBS. Therefore, individual responses and experiences may vary. It is always best to work with a healthcare professional who can provide guidance tailored to your unique needs and circumstances.

Intermittent fasting is an eating pattern that involves cycling between periods of fasting and eating within a designated timeframe. While some individuals with Irritable Bowel Syndrome (IBS) may find intermittent fasting beneficial, it's important to approach it with caution and consider individual factors. Here are some points to consider regarding intermittent fasting and IBS:

1. Individual Variability: Responses to intermittent fasting can vary among individuals with IBS. Some people may find that adopting an intermittent fasting schedule helps regulate their eating patterns, reduces bloating, and improves symptoms. However, others may experience increased symptoms or discomfort during fasting periods. It's

essential to listen to your body and assess how intermittent fasting affects your IBS symptoms.

2. Impact on Meal Timing: Intermittent fasting typically involves restricting the eating window, which may affect meal timing. For individuals with IBS, maintaining regular meal patterns and avoiding long periods without food may help manage symptoms. Consider whether intermittent fasting aligns with your personal meal preferences and if it supports your digestive well-being.

3. Nutritional Adequacy: It's important to ensure that your meals during the eating window provide adequate nutrition. Focus on consuming a balanced diet with a variety of nutrient-rich foods, including fruits, vegetables, whole grains, lean proteins, and healthy fats. If you're following a specific diet plan or have dietary restrictions, consult with a registered dietitian to ensure your nutritional needs are met.

4. Impact on Gut Motility: Changes in meal timing and fasting periods may impact gut motility and digestion. Some individuals with IBS may experience changes in bowel movements or increased symptoms during fasting periods. Assess how your body responds to intermittent fasting and if it affects your digestion or triggers symptoms.

5. Consideration of Stress and Emotional Factors: Intermittent fasting may cause additional stress or anxiety around food and eating patterns, particularly for individuals with a strong psychological component to their IBS symptoms. Be mindful of your emotional well-being and ensure that intermittent fasting doesn't exacerbate stress levels, as stress can influence IBS symptoms.

As with any dietary approach, it is recommended to consult with a healthcare professional, such as a registered dietitian or gastroenterologist, who is knowledgeable about IBS and your specific medical history. They can provide personalized guidance, taking into account your individual needs and symptoms, and help determine if intermittent fasting is suitable for you. Additionally, keeping a food diary to track your symptoms and responses to intermittent fasting can be helpful in understanding how it affects your IBS.

IBS MEDITATION

Meditation can be a beneficial practice for individuals with Irritable Bowel Syndrome (IBS) as it promotes relaxation, stress reduction, and overall well-being. Here are some ways in which meditation can potentially help manage IBS:

1. Stress Reduction: Stress is known to exacerbate IBS symptoms. Engaging in regular meditation practice can help reduce stress levels and promote a sense of calmness and relaxation. By cultivating a relaxed state of mind, you may experience a reduction in IBS symptoms triggered by stress.
2. Mind-Body Connection: Meditation can help foster a stronger mind-body connection, allowing you to become more aware of the sensations, emotions, and triggers associated with your IBS. This increased awareness can empower you to better understand and manage your symptoms.
3. Pain Management: Mindfulness meditation techniques can be effective in managing pain, including abdominal pain and discomfort associated with IBS. By bringing focused attention to the present moment and adopting a non-judgmental attitude toward pain sensations, you may experience a reduction in pain perception.
4. Emotional Regulation: IBS can be influenced by emotions such as anxiety, frustration, and fear. Meditation practices, such as loving-kindness meditation or compassion meditation, can cultivate positive emotions and improve emotional regulation, potentially reducing the impact of emotions on IBS symptoms.
5. Improved Sleep: IBS symptoms can disrupt sleep, and poor sleep quality can, in turn, worsen IBS symptoms. Engaging

in meditation before bedtime can help calm the mind, relax the body, and promote better sleep, leading to improved overall well-being.

Here are a few meditation techniques that may be beneficial for individuals with IBS:

- Mindfulness Meditation: Focus on the present moment, observe your thoughts, emotions, and bodily sensations without judgment, and gently bring your attention back to the breath or a chosen focal point.
- Body Scan Meditation: Bring attention to different parts of your body, noticing any sensations or areas of tension, and allowing them to relax with each breath.
- Loving-Kindness Meditation: Cultivate feelings of compassion, love, and kindness toward yourself and others, which can help reduce stress and foster a positive emotional state.
- Guided Imagery Meditation: Visualize calming and soothing scenes or environments, such as a peaceful beach or a tranquil forest, to induce relaxation and alleviate stress.

It's important to note that meditation is a practice that requires consistency and patience. You may find it helpful to start with shorter sessions and gradually increase the duration as you become more comfortable. If you're new to meditation, there are numerous smartphone apps, online resources, and guided meditation recordings available that can provide guidance and support.

As always, it's recommended to consult with healthcare professionals, such as psychologists or mindfulness instructors, who can provide further guidance and tailor the meditation practices to your specific needs and preferences.

IBS INTENSIVE TRAINING

Engaging in intensive sport training while living with Irritable Bowel Syndrome (IBS) requires careful consideration and management. While some individuals with IBS may be able to participate in intense physical activity without significant issues, others may find that certain aspects of intensive training can trigger or worsen their symptoms. Here are some factors to consider when engaging in intensive sport training with IBS:

1. Individual Variability: Responses to intense exercise can vary among individuals with IBS. Some people may experience symptom relief or improved bowel regularity during and after exercise, while others may find that intense physical activity triggers or exacerbates their symptoms. It's important to pay attention to your body and understand how different types and intensities of exercise affect your symptoms.

2. Impact of Stress and Anxiety: Intensive training can be physically and mentally demanding, potentially leading to increased stress and anxiety levels. For individuals with IBS, stress and anxiety are known triggers for symptom flare-ups. It's essential to find ways to manage and reduce stress during training, such as incorporating relaxation techniques or mindfulness practices.

3. Hydration and Nutrition: Intensive training requires proper hydration and nutrition. For individuals with IBS, it may be necessary to pay attention to specific dietary triggers and ensure that pre- and post-training meals are well-tolerated and support optimal performance. Working with a registered dietitian who is knowledgeable about sports nutrition and IBS can help you develop an individualized plan.

4. Impact on Digestive System: Intense physical activity can affect gut motility and potentially lead to digestive symptoms. Some individuals with IBS may experience increased abdominal pain, bloating, or changes in bowel movements during or after training. It's important to be aware of these potential triggers and consider modifying your training routine accordingly.

5. Rest and Recovery: Intensive training requires adequate rest and recovery periods. Overtraining or insufficient rest can increase stress on the body, potentially worsening IBS symptoms. Ensure that your training program incorporates sufficient rest days and prioritize recovery strategies such as proper sleep, stretching, and relaxation techniques.

6. Seek Professional Guidance: If you plan to engage in intensive sport training with IBS, it's advisable to consult with healthcare professionals, including a gastroenterologist and a sports medicine specialist. They can provide personalized advice, evaluate your specific condition and needs, and help develop a training plan that takes into account your IBS symptoms and limitations.

Pay attention to your body, communicate with your healthcare team, and make necessary adjustments to your training routine to manage your symptoms effectively and support your overall well-being.

Rowing can be a suitable form of exercise for individuals with Irritable Bowel Syndrome (IBS) as it is a low-impact, full-body workout that can be tailored to different fitness levels. However, it's important to consider certain factors when incorporating rowing into your routine if you have IBS:

1. Individual Tolerance: Every person with IBS may have different responses to exercise, including rowing. Some

individuals may find that rowing helps alleviate their symptoms, while others may experience symptom exacerbation. Monitor your body's response to rowing and adjust the intensity and duration based on your comfort level.

2. Impact on Digestive System: Intense exercise, including rowing, can potentially affect gut motility and lead to digestive symptoms. Some individuals with IBS may experience increased abdominal discomfort, bloating, or changes in bowel movements during or after rowing. It's important to be aware of these potential triggers and consider modifying your rowing routine accordingly.

3. Hydration and Nutrition: Proper hydration and nutrition are important when engaging in physical activity like rowing. Ensure that you are adequately hydrated before, during, and after rowing sessions. If certain foods or specific dietary triggers worsen your symptoms, pay attention to your pre- and post-workout meals to ensure they are well-tolerated.

4. Stress Management: Intense exercise can be physically and mentally demanding, potentially leading to increased stress and anxiety levels. Stress is known to trigger or worsen IBS symptoms. Incorporate stress management techniques such as deep breathing, mindfulness, or meditation to help manage stress during your rowing sessions.

5. Gradual Progression: If you are new to rowing or have been inactive for a while, it's important to start gradually and progress slowly. Sudden intense workouts may put additional stress on your body and potentially exacerbate your symptoms. Begin with shorter sessions and gradually increase the duration and intensity of your rowing workouts as your body adapts.

6. Personalized Approach: Each person with IBS is unique, and what works for one may not work for another. Listen to

your body, communicate with your healthcare team, and make adjustments to your rowing routine based on your symptoms and comfort level. It may be beneficial to consult with a sports medicine specialist or a physical therapist who can provide guidance on proper technique and modifications.

Remember to prioritize rest, recovery, and self-care in your overall fitness routine. This includes getting sufficient sleep, incorporating stretching and relaxation techniques, and allowing for adequate recovery time between rowing sessions.

As always, it's important to consult with your healthcare provider, especially if you have any specific medical concerns or if you are unsure about the suitability of rowing or any other form of exercise for your individual condition. They can provide personalized advice and guidance tailored to your needs.

IBS ANIMALS

Animals, particularly trained therapy animals, can play a supportive role in managing symptoms and improving well-being for individuals with various health conditions, including Irritable Bowel Syndrome (IBS). Here are some ways in which animals can potentially contribute to IBS management:

1. Emotional Support: Animals, such as therapy dogs or cats, can provide emotional support and companionship. The presence of a supportive animal can help reduce stress, anxiety, and feelings of isolation, which may be beneficial for individuals with IBS who experience symptom flare-ups triggered by stress.
2. Stress Reduction: Interacting with animals has been shown to reduce stress and promote relaxation. Petting or spending time with animals can release endorphins, which can have a positive effect on mood and overall well-being. Stress reduction can be particularly important for managing IBS symptoms, as stress is known to exacerbate symptoms.
3. Distraction and Comfort: Animals can provide a distraction from IBS symptoms and offer comfort during times of discomfort or pain. The presence of a beloved pet can help shift focus away from symptoms and provide a sense of comfort and support.
4. Routine and Responsibility: Taking care of an animal can provide a sense of routine and responsibility, which can be beneficial for individuals with IBS. Establishing a consistent routine, such as feeding or walking a pet, can help individuals with IBS maintain regularity in their daily activities.
5. Increased Physical Activity: Owning a dog, for example, can encourage regular physical activity through walks or

playtime. Engaging in moderate exercise can have positive effects on digestion, bowel regularity, and overall well-being for individuals with IBS.

It's important to note that the suitability of having an animal companion or therapy animal for IBS management can vary depending on individual preferences, allergies, and living situations. If considering a therapy animal, it's advisable to consult with a healthcare professional or therapist who can provide guidance on the potential benefits and help determine if it's a suitable option for you.

Additionally, it's essential to ensure proper care, training, and attention to the needs of any animal companion. Consider factors such as allergies, time commitment, and financial responsibility before making a decision.

Overall, while animals can provide emotional support, comfort, and potential health benefits, it's important to incorporate a comprehensive approach to managing IBS symptoms, which may include lifestyle modifications, medical treatments, and support from healthcare professionals.

IBS MASSAGE

Massage therapy can be a complementary approach to managing the symptoms of Irritable Bowel Syndrome (IBS). While it may not directly treat the underlying causes of IBS, massage can provide relaxation, stress reduction, and potential relief from certain symptoms. Here are some ways in which massage therapy may be beneficial for individuals with IBS:

1. Stress Reduction: Massage therapy promotes relaxation and helps reduce stress and anxiety. Since stress can trigger or exacerbate IBS symptoms, receiving regular massages can help create a more calm and relaxed state of mind, potentially leading to a reduction in symptom severity.
2. Improved Digestion and Bowel Function: Massage techniques, such as abdominal massage or lymphatic drainage, can stimulate the digestive system and help improve bowel function. It can enhance blood circulation, ease muscle tension, and potentially relieve symptoms such as bloating, cramping, and constipation.
3. Pain Relief: Some individuals with IBS experience abdominal pain or discomfort. Massage therapy can help alleviate muscle tension, release endorphins (natural pain relievers), and provide temporary relief from pain associated with IBS.
4. Enhanced Body Awareness: Massage therapy can help individuals become more aware of their body, including areas of tension or discomfort. This increased body awareness can empower individuals to better manage their symptoms and make necessary adjustments to their daily routines and self-care practices.
5. Relaxation Response: Massage therapy activates the parasympathetic nervous system, triggering the body's

relaxation response. This can lead to a decrease in heart rate, blood pressure, and stress hormone levels, promoting a sense of overall well-being and potentially reducing the impact of stress on IBS symptoms.

It's important to note that the effectiveness of massage therapy for IBS can vary from person to person. It's recommended to work with a licensed and experienced massage therapist who understands the unique considerations of IBS and can tailor the massage techniques to your specific needs and comfort level.

While massage therapy can provide potential benefits, it is not a substitute for medical treatment or other lifestyle modifications. It's advisable to consult with your healthcare provider or gastroenterologist to discuss incorporating massage therapy into your overall management plan for IBS. They can provide guidance on whether massage therapy is suitable for you and how it can be integrated into your comprehensive approach to managing IBS symptoms.

IBS SEX AND LOVE

Irritable bowel syndrome (IBS) is a medical condition that primarily affects the gastrointestinal system, causing symptoms such as abdominal pain, bloating, diarrhea, and constipation. It is not directly related to sexual health or sexual activity.

However, it's important to note that IBS can have an impact on various aspects of a person's life, including their emotional well-being and intimate relationships. Individuals with IBS may experience changes in their sexual function and libido due to factors such as pain, discomfort, or anxiety related to their condition.

If you are experiencing challenges in your sexual health or intimate relationships due to IBS, it's important to discuss these concerns with a healthcare professional. They can provide guidance and support tailored to your specific situation. They may also be able to help identify strategies or treatments that can alleviate symptoms and improve your overall quality of life, which can indirectly have a positive impact on your sexual well-being.

Remember, open communication with your healthcare provider is key to addressing any concerns or challenges you may be facing. They can provide appropriate advice and support to help you navigate the impact of IBS on your sexual health.

Living with Irritable Bowel Syndrome (IBS) can undoubtedly present challenges, but it's important to remember that having IBS does not diminish your ability to experience and cultivate love in your life. Here are some thoughts on love and managing IBS:

1. Self-Love and Acceptance: Practicing self-love and acceptance is crucial when living with any chronic condition, including IBS. Embrace yourself, including your body and your experiences, and cultivate a compassionate and nurturing relationship with yourself.
2. Supportive Relationships: Surround yourself with supportive and understanding people who love and accept you for who you are, including your experiences with IBS. Openly communicate with your loved ones about your condition, educate them about IBS, and let them provide the support and understanding you need.
3. Emotional Connection: Love is not solely defined by physical aspects but also by emotional connection. Focus on nurturing emotional intimacy in your relationships. Share your thoughts, feelings, and concerns with your partner, family, or friends. Building strong emotional bonds can help create a loving and supportive environment.
4. Open Communication: Open communication is essential in any relationship, especially when it comes to managing IBS. Be open and honest about your symptoms, triggers, and limitations. Discuss your needs, such as flexibility with plans or understanding during flare-ups. A loving and supportive partner will be willing to adapt and accommodate your needs.
5. Intimacy and Sensuality: IBS may present challenges when it comes to physical intimacy, but it doesn't mean that love and intimacy are impossible. Engage in open and honest conversations with your partner about your comfort level, triggers, and ways to enjoy physical intimacy without exacerbating symptoms. Explore alternative forms of intimacy that focus on emotional connection and closeness.
6. Managing Stress: Stress can worsen IBS symptoms and impact your overall well-being. Prioritize stress

management techniques, such as meditation, relaxation exercises, or engaging in activities you enjoy. By managing stress, you create a more loving and harmonious environment for yourself and those around you.

7. Seeking Professional Help: If you are experiencing difficulties in relationships or struggling with the emotional impact of IBS, consider seeking professional help. A therapist or counselor can provide guidance and support in navigating relationship challenges and emotional well-being.

Remember, love is not limited by your condition. IBS may present challenges, but it doesn't define you or your ability to give and receive love. Embrace self-love, build supportive relationships, communicate openly, and seek the understanding and compassion you deserve. With love, understanding, and acceptance, it's possible to cultivate fulfilling and loving connections in your life, despite living with IBS.

It's important to approach the management of Irritable Bowel Syndrome (IBS) with a balanced and holistic mindset. While it's natural to desire control over your symptoms, enforcing aggressive control may not be the most effective approach. Here are some considerations:

1. Gentle Approach: Instead of enforcing aggressive control, consider adopting a gentle approach to managing your symptoms. Focus on self-care, stress reduction, and making gradual changes to your lifestyle and diet. Aggressive control measures may increase stress levels and potentially worsen symptoms.

2. Individual Variability: Each person with IBS may have different triggers and sensitivities. What works for one person may not work for another. It's important to be

patient and experiment with different strategies to find what works best for you. Collaborating with a healthcare professional, such as a gastroenterologist or registered dietitian, can provide personalized guidance.

3. Lifestyle Modifications: Implementing lifestyle modifications can play a significant role in managing IBS symptoms. This includes incorporating regular physical activity, practicing stress reduction techniques (e.g., mindfulness, meditation), and prioritizing restful sleep. These gentle adjustments can have a positive impact on your overall well-being.

4. Dietary Modifications: Making changes to your diet can be beneficial, but it's important to approach it in a balanced manner. Consider exploring a low-FODMAP diet or other dietary modifications under the guidance of a registered dietitian. They can help you identify trigger foods and develop a sustainable and individualized eating plan.

5. Emotional Well-being: Aggressive control may lead to increased stress, anxiety, and frustration. It's important to prioritize your emotional well-being and seek support when needed. Engaging in activities that promote relaxation, practicing self-compassion, and seeking counseling or therapy can be beneficial.

6. Medications and Treatments: If lifestyle and dietary modifications are not sufficient, consult with your healthcare provider about medical treatments for IBS. They can assess your specific symptoms and recommend appropriate medications or therapies to help manage your symptoms effectively.

7. Support Network: Building a support network of understanding friends, family, or support groups can provide emotional support and a sense of community. Sharing experiences, seeking advice, and learning from others who have similar challenges can be empowering.

Remember, enforcing aggressive control over your symptoms may lead to frustration and disappointment. It's important to find a balance between actively managing your condition and allowing yourself some flexibility and self-compassion. Collaborating with healthcare professionals, practicing self-care, and seeking support from loved ones can help you navigate the challenges of IBS in a healthier and more sustainable way.

Sexual arousal and orgasm can potentially have an impact on the symptoms of Irritable Bowel Syndrome (IBS) for some individuals. Here are some points to consider:

1. Relaxation and Stress Reduction: Sexual arousal and orgasm can promote relaxation and release endorphins, which are natural pain-relieving and mood-enhancing chemicals. This relaxation response may help temporarily alleviate stress and reduce the impact of stress on IBS symptoms.
2. Physical Stimulation: Some individuals may experience relief from certain gastrointestinal symptoms, such as abdominal pain or cramping, during sexual activity. This may be due to the physical stimulation and release of tension in the pelvic area.
3. Individual Variability: The impact of sexual arousal and orgasm on IBS symptoms can vary among individuals. While some may experience temporary relief or even improved symptom management, others may find that sexual activity can trigger or worsen their symptoms. It's important to listen to your body and assess how sexual activity affects your symptoms.
4. Emotional and Psychological Factors: Emotional and psychological factors can play a significant role in IBS symptoms. For some individuals, positive emotional experiences, such as intimacy and connection during sexual

activity, can have a beneficial impact on overall well-being and potentially improve IBS symptoms.

5. Communication and Consent: It's essential to prioritize open communication and consent in any sexual activity. Communicate your needs, concerns, and comfort levels with your partner to ensure a safe and enjoyable experience that takes into account your specific IBS symptoms and limitations.

It's important to note that sexual activity, including orgasm, is a personal and intimate experience. It may not be suitable or comfortable for everyone, depending on their individual circumstances and symptoms. If you have specific concerns or questions about the impact of sexual activity on your IBS symptoms, it's recommended to consult with your healthcare provider or gastroenterologist, who can provide personalized advice and guidance based on your unique situation.

Overall, understanding your body, communicating with your partner, and being attentive to your physical and emotional well-being can help you navigate the impact of sexual arousal and orgasm on your IBS symptoms.

IBS JOBS AND CAREER

Irritable bowel syndrome (IBS) is a medical condition that affects the gastrointestinal system, causing symptoms such as abdominal pain, bloating, and changes in bowel habits. While IBS can impact a person's daily life, it does not specifically limit or determine the type of job a person can pursue.

Individuals with IBS can have a wide range of career options depending on their skills, qualifications, and personal preferences. It's important to consider your individual symptoms, triggers, and needs when selecting a job or career path. Here are a few factors to keep in mind:

Flexibility: Consider jobs that offer flexible working hours or the ability to work from home when necessary. This can help accommodate any unpredictable symptoms or flare-ups associated with IBS.

Stress Management: Some individuals with IBS find that high-stress environments can worsen their symptoms. It may be beneficial to seek job roles that offer a lower-stress work environment or positions that allow for stress management techniques such as mindfulness or relaxation exercises.

Physical Demands: Depending on the severity of your symptoms, it may be helpful to assess the physical demands of a job. Some individuals with IBS may find it challenging to engage in physically strenuous or demanding work. Considering job roles that are less physically demanding or have accommodations for physical limitations can be beneficial.

Supportive Work Environment: Look for companies or workplaces that prioritize employee well-being and offer support systems such as Employee Assistance Programs (EAPs) or accommodations for individuals with chronic health conditions.

Ultimately, it's important to find a job that aligns with your skills, interests, and accommodates your individual needs. Discussing your specific situation and any work-related concerns with a healthcare professional or career counselor may provide further guidance and support in finding the right job for you.

IBS SLEEP

Getting sufficient and restful sleep is essential for overall well-being, and it can have a significant impact on managing symptoms of Irritable Bowel Syndrome (IBS). Here are some considerations regarding sleep and IBS:

1. Sleep Hygiene: Prioritize good sleep hygiene practices to promote better sleep. Establish a consistent sleep schedule by going to bed and waking up at the same time each day, even on weekends. Create a comfortable sleep environment that is cool, dark, and quiet. Avoid stimulating activities and electronic devices before bed, and engage in relaxing activities to signal your body that it's time to sleep.
2. Symptom Management: Addressing IBS symptoms that can disrupt sleep, such as abdominal pain, bloating, or frequent bowel movements, can help improve sleep quality. Work with your healthcare provider to develop an effective management plan for your specific symptoms, including dietary modifications, medications, stress reduction techniques, and other strategies.
3. Diet and Bedtime Snacks: Be mindful of your diet and the timing of meals and snacks, particularly before bed. Large or heavy meals close to bedtime can disrupt sleep. Consider avoiding trigger foods that may worsen your symptoms before sleep, and opt for lighter, easily digestible snacks if needed.
4. Stress Reduction: High stress levels can impact both sleep quality and IBS symptoms. Incorporate stress reduction techniques into your daily routine, such as relaxation exercises, meditation, or deep breathing. Establishing a bedtime routine that includes calming activities can help

transition your body and mind into a relaxed state for
sleep.
5. Physical Activity: Regular physical activity can help promote
    better sleep. Engage in moderate exercise during the day,
    but avoid intense workouts close to bedtime, as they may
    interfere with sleep. Find a balance that works for you and
    your individual symptoms.
6. Sleep Disorders: If you suspect you may have a sleep
    disorder, such as insomnia or sleep apnea, it's important to
    seek evaluation and treatment from a healthcare
    professional. Addressing any underlying sleep disorders can
    significantly improve sleep quality and overall well-being.
7. Consult with Healthcare Professionals: If you are
    experiencing persistent sleep difficulties related to IBS or if
    sleep disturbances significantly impact your quality of life,
    consult with your healthcare provider. They can provide
    personalized guidance, evaluate any potential underlying
    factors contributing to sleep problems, and recommend
    appropriate interventions.

Remember that everyone's sleep needs and patterns are unique. It
may take time and experimentation to find what works best for
you. Prioritizing sleep as an integral part of your overall wellness
routine can contribute to better management of IBS symptoms
and improved quality of life.

RESOURCES

Here is a list of 10 resources related to Irritable Bowel Syndrome (IBS):

1. International Foundation for Functional Gastrointestinal Disorders (IFFGD) - Provides comprehensive information on IBS, treatment options, and support resources. Website: https://www.iffgd.org/
2. The American Gastroenterological Association (AGA) - Offers patient education materials and resources on IBS diagnosis and management. Website: https://gastro.org/
3. The Rome Foundation - A nonprofit organization that provides educational resources and clinical guidelines for functional gastrointestinal disorders, including IBS. Website: https://theromefoundation.org/
4. National Institute of Diabetes and Digestive and Kidney Diseases (NIDDK) - Part of the National Institutes of Health (NIH), NIDDK offers educational materials, research updates, and clinical trial information on IBS. Website: https://www.niddk.nih.gov/
5. IBS Impact - A nonprofit organization dedicated to raising awareness and providing support for individuals with IBS. Their website includes resources, personal stories, and links to IBS communities. Website: https://www.ibsimpact.com/
6. Monash University - Provides valuable information on the low-FODMAP diet, including food lists, recipes, and research updates. Website: https://www.monashfodmap.com/
7. The American College of Gastroenterology (ACG) - Offers patient information on IBS diagnosis and management. Website: https://gi.org/

8. IBS Network - A UK-based charity that supports individuals with IBS, providing resources, information, and a helpline. Website: https://www.theibsnetwork.org/
9. Healthline - Offers comprehensive articles, guides, and resources on IBS symptoms, causes, and management strategies. Website: https://www.healthline.com/health/ibs
10. Mayo Clinic - Provides reliable information on IBS symptoms, diagnosis, and treatment options. Website: https://www.mayoclinic.org/

Please note that this list is not exhaustive, and it's always a good idea to consult with healthcare professionals and trusted sources for accurate and up-to-date information on IBS.

Here is a list of 10 YouTube channels that provide valuable information and resources related to Irritable Bowel Syndrome (IBS):

1. Monash University FODMAP - Official channel of Monash University, known for their research on the low-FODMAP diet and IBS. They provide educational videos, cooking tutorials, and updates on the latest research: https://www.youtube.com/user/MonashFODMAP
2. The IBS Academy - Provides educational videos on IBS management, including tips for symptom relief, dietary advice, and lifestyle strategies: https://www.youtube.com/c/TheIBSAcademy
3. Dr. Jocelyn Strand - A gastroenterologist who shares informative videos on IBS, including diagnosis, treatment options, and dietary recommendations: https://www.youtube.com/c/DrJocelynStrand

4. The IBS Solution - Offers videos on IBS triggers, symptom management, and tips for living well with IBS: https://www.youtube.com/c/TheIBSSolution

5. Gastrointestinal Society - Covers various digestive health topics, including IBS, with videos featuring healthcare professionals and patient stories: https://www.youtube.com/user/gastrointestinalbc

6. The Mind-Gut Connection - Dr. Emeran Mayer, a leading expert on the gut-brain connection, explores the relationship between the gut and brain and its impact on conditions like IBS: https://www.youtube.com/c/TheMindGutConnection

7. FODMAP Life - Provides videos on the low-FODMAP diet, cooking tips, and recipe ideas for individuals with IBS and other digestive disorders: https://www.youtube.com/c/FODMAPLife

8. Healthy Gut - Dr. Michael Ruscio discusses gut health topics, including IBS, gut microbiome, and evidence-based approaches to managing digestive disorders: https://www.youtube.com/user/drmichaelruscio

9. Everyday Health - Offers a wide range of videos on health topics, including IBS, with interviews, expert advice, and lifestyle tips: https://www.youtube.com/c/EverydayHealth

10. Mayo Clinic - Provides videos on various health conditions, including IBS, with expert insights, treatment options, and patient stories: https://www.youtube.com/user/mayoclinic

These channels offer valuable insights and resources for individuals seeking information and support regarding IBS. Remember to always consult with healthcare professionals for personalized advice and guidance in managing your specific condition.

Here is a list of 10 blogs that provide informative content and resources related to Irritable Bowel Syndrome (IBS):

1. Kate Scarlata - Kate Scarlata is a registered dietitian and author who specializes in digestive health, including IBS. Her blog offers educational articles, low-FODMAP recipes, and tips for managing IBS: https://www.katescarlata.com/blog/

2. The Gut Health Doctor - Dr. Megan Rossi, a registered dietitian and gut health expert, shares evidence-based information on IBS and digestive health on her blog: https://www.theguthealthdoctor.com/blog/

3. A Little Bit Yummy - Provides a collection of low-FODMAP recipes, meal plans, and articles to support individuals with IBS on their journey to manage symptoms and enjoy flavorful food: https://alittlebityummy.com/blog/

4. The IBS Diaries - Written by a personal IBS sufferer, this blog offers insights, experiences, and tips for managing IBS symptoms and living a fulfilling life: https://theibsdiaries.com/

5. The Well Balanced FODMAPer - A blog dedicated to the low-FODMAP diet, offering recipes, meal ideas, and practical tips for navigating life with IBS: https://www.wellbalancedfodmaper.com/blog

6. The Belly Rules the Mind - Focuses on gut health and provides recipes, meal plans, and lifestyle tips for individuals with IBS and other digestive conditions: https://thebellyrulesthemind.net/

7. My Gut Feeling - Offers low-FODMAP recipes, tips for dining out with IBS, and personal stories from the author's journey with IBS: https://www.mygutfeeling.eu/

8. The Reluctant Spoonie - A blog that addresses life with chronic illness, including IBS, providing relatable stories, tips for self-care, and navigating the ups and downs of living with a chronic condition: https://thereluctantspoonie.com/

9. A Gutsy Girl - Covers various digestive health topics, including IBS, with articles on gut health, lifestyle, and personal experiences: https://agutsygirl.com/
10. Low FODMAP Journey - Offers information and resources on the low-FODMAP diet, including recipes, meal plans, and tips for managing IBS symptoms: https://www.lowfodmapjourney.com/blog/

These blogs provide a wealth of information, personal stories, and practical tips for managing IBS symptoms and living well with the condition. Remember to consult with healthcare professionals for personalized advice and guidance in managing your specific situation.

Here is a list of 10 highly regarded books that provide valuable information and insights on Irritable Bowel Syndrome (IBS):

1. "The Complete Low-FODMAP Diet: A Revolutionary Plan for Managing IBS and Other Digestive Disorders" by Sue Shepherd and Peter Gibson.
   o This comprehensive guidebook provides information on the low-FODMAP diet, including recipes, meal plans, and strategies for managing IBS symptoms.
2. "The IBS Elimination Diet and Cookbook: The Proven Low-FODMAP Plan for Eating Well and Feeling Great" by Patsy Catsos.
   o This book offers an elimination diet approach to managing IBS through the low-FODMAP diet, along with a collection of delicious recipes and practical tips.
3. "IBS for Dummies" by Carolyn Dean and L. Christine Wheeler.

- A beginner-friendly guide that covers various aspects of IBS, including symptoms, diagnosis, treatment options, and lifestyle strategies for managing the condition.

4. "The Mind-Gut Connection: How the Hidden Conversation Within Our Bodies Impacts Our Mood, Our Choices, and Our Overall Health" by Emeran Mayer.
   - Explores the complex relationship between the gut and the brain, providing insights into the gut-brain connection and its impact on conditions like IBS.

5. "The IBS Healing Plan: Natural Ways to Beat Your Symptoms" by Theresa Cheung.
   - Offers a holistic approach to managing IBS, combining natural remedies, lifestyle adjustments, and dietary strategies to alleviate symptoms and improve overall well-being.

6. "IBS (Irritable Bowel Syndrome) and GI Solutions: The Ultimate Guide to Achieving Relief from IBS and Other Digestive Disorders" by Dr. Mark Pimentel.
   - Written by a leading expert in the field, this book provides comprehensive information on IBS, treatment options, and innovative approaches to managing the condition.

7. "The First Year: IBS (Irritable Bowel Syndrome): An Essential Guide for the Newly Diagnosed" by Heather Van Vorous.
   - Aimed at individuals recently diagnosed with IBS, this book offers practical advice, tips for symptom management, and strategies for coping with the challenges of living with the condition.

8. "Eating for IBS: 175 Delicious, Nutritious, Low-FODMAP Recipes to Stabilize the Gut and Manage Symptoms of IBS" by Heather Van Vorous.
   - Focuses on providing flavorful and nutritious recipes that align with the low-FODMAP diet,

offering options for individuals with IBS to enjoy delicious meals while managing their symptoms.

9. "IBS Chat: Real Life Stories and Solutions" by Barbara Bolen and Kathleen Bradley.
    - Features real-life stories from individuals with IBS, along with practical tips, coping strategies, and insights from healthcare professionals.
10. "The Second Brain: A Groundbreaking New Understanding of Nervous Disorders of the Stomach and Intestine" by Michael Gershon.

- Explores the concept of the "second brain" residing in the gut, shedding light on the intricate connection between the gut and the central nervous system, with relevance to conditions like IBS.

These books offer a range of perspectives, strategies, and insights into managing IBS. It's important to note that individual experiences and needs may vary, so it's always recommended to consult with healthcare professionals for personalized advice and guidance in managing your specific condition.

Here are some prominent IBS-related associations and organizations that provide resources, support, and information on IBS:

1. International Foundation for Functional Gastrointestinal Disorders (IFFGD) - Based in the United States, IFFGD is a nonprofit organization that provides educational resources, support groups, research updates, and advocacy for individuals with gastrointestinal disorders, including IBS. Website: https://www.iffgd.org/
2. The Rome Foundation - An international nonprofit organization focused on the diagnosis and management of

functional gastrointestinal disorders, including IBS. They provide clinical guidelines, research, and educational resources. Website: https://theromefoundation.org/

3. The IBS Network - A UK-based charity that supports individuals with IBS through information, resources, helpline services, and local support groups. Website: https://www.theibsnetwork.org/

4. Gastrointestinal Society - A Canadian nonprofit organization that provides educational resources, support, and advocacy for individuals with digestive disorders, including IBS. Website: https://www.badgut.org/

5. IBS Impact - A US-based nonprofit organization that aims to raise awareness, provide support, and advocate for individuals with IBS. They offer resources, personal stories, and links to IBS communities. Website: https://www.ibsimpact.com/

6. Australian Centre for Functional Gut Disorders (ACFGD) - An Australian organization that focuses on education, research, and support for individuals with functional gut disorders, including IBS. Website: https://acfgd.com.au/

7. Canadian Society of Intestinal Research (CSIR) - A Canadian organization that provides information, research updates, and support for individuals with intestinal disorders, including IBS. Website: https://badgut.org/

8. German Society for Neurogastroenterology and Motility (DGNM) - A German association that focuses on research, education, and the promotion of knowledge in the field of neurogastroenterology and motility disorders, including IBS. Website: https://www.dgnm.de/

9. IBS Network Australia - An Australian organization that offers support, education, and advocacy for individuals with IBS, including online resources, support groups, and community engagement. Website: https://ibs-network.org/

10. International Foundation for Gastrointestinal Disorders
    (IFFGD) - Based in the United States, this foundation
    focuses on promoting awareness, advocacy, research, and
    support for individuals with gastrointestinal disorders,
    including IBS. Website: https://iffgd.org/

While this list provides a starting point, it is always recommended
to search for local IBS associations or support groups specific to
your country or region for more localized resources and support.
Additionally, healthcare professionals or gastroenterology
associations in your country may also provide resources and
information on IBS.

FINAL THOUGHTS

Living with Irritable Bowel Syndrome (IBS) can be challenging, but it's important to remember that you are not alone. With proper management strategies, support, and a positive mindset, it is possible to lead a fulfilling life while effectively managing your symptoms.

Remember to be patient and kind to yourself. Finding the right combination of treatments, lifestyle adjustments, and self-care practices may take time, so don't get discouraged if you experience setbacks along the way. Each person's journey with IBS is unique, and what works for one may not work for another. Stay open-minded and willing to explore different approaches until you find what works best for you.

Seeking support from healthcare professionals, support groups, or online communities can be invaluable. Surround yourself with understanding and compassionate individuals who can offer encouragement, share experiences, and provide helpful advice.

Maintaining a balanced and healthy lifestyle is crucial. Focus on self-care activities that promote relaxation, stress reduction, and overall well-being. Practice mindfulness, engage in regular physical activity, get adequate sleep, and nourish your body with a balanced diet.

Finally, stay positive and keep a hopeful outlook. While IBS may present challenges, it doesn't define you. Your strength, resilience, and determination to manage your symptoms and live a fulfilling life are commendable. Remember to celebrate small victories along the way and acknowledge the progress you've made.

Keep moving forward, and remember that you have the ability to overcome the challenges of IBS and live a meaningful and satisfying life. You are not defined by your condition, but by the strength and resilience you demonstrate in managing it. Stay hopeful, take one step at a time, and believe in your ability to create a fulfilling life despite the obstacles you may face.